Physical Therapy and the Stroke Patient: Pathologic Aspects and Clinical Management

Physical Therapy and the Stroke Patient: Pathologic Aspects and Clinical Management

Mary C. Singleton and Eleanor F. Branch
Co-Editors

The Haworth Press
New York • London

MT

Physical Therapy and the Stroke Patient: Pathologic Aspects and Clinical Management has also been published as *Physical Therapy in Health Care*, Volume 1, Number 4, Summer 1987.

The Haworth Press, Inc., 12 West 32 Street, New York, NY 10001
EUROSPAN/Haworth, 3 Henrietta Street, London WC2E 8LU England

Library of Congress Cataloging-in-Publication Data

Physical therapy and the stroke patient.
  "Has also been published as Physical therapy in health care, vol. 1 (4), summer 1987" — T.p. verso.
  Includes bibliographies.
    1. Cerebrovascular disease — Patients — Rehabilitation. 2. Physical therapy. I. Singleton, Mary C. II. Branch, Eleanor F. [DNLM: 1. Cerebrovascular Disorders — physiopathology. 2. Cerebrovascular Disorders — rehabilitation. 3. Physical Therapy — methods.
W1 PH749JE v.1 no.4 / WL 355 P578
RC388.5.P48 1987   616.8'1   87-26668
ISBN 0-86656-740-2

Physical Therapy and the Stroke Patient: Pathologic Aspects and Clinical Management

Physical Therapy in Health Care
Volume 1, Number 4

CONTENTS

Foreword

This issue of *Physical Therapy in Health Care* focuses on the subject of cerebrovascular accidents. Physical therapists are key health professionals in the care of the stroke patient; it is essential, therefore, that they be cognizant of the pathologic and clinical features of common ischemic and hemorrhagic disorders that may culminate in the familiar signs and symptoms of stroke. Such knowledge should serve as a challenge and impetus to the ingenuity and creativity of therapists as they approach the management of a group of patients commonly encountered in general hospital, nursing home, and rehabilitation settings. The editors trust that the reader will come away with an appreciation of the variability of involvement among stroke patients and, therefore, will approach their management in an individualistic manner.

Physical Therapy and the Stroke Patient: Pathologic Aspects and Clinical Management

Diagnostic, Medical, and Surgical Approaches to Stroke Management

E. Wayne Massey, MD

SUMMARY. Hemorrhagic and ischemic brain damage causing stroke ranks third among the causes of death in the United States. The evaluation of patients with stroke must be extensive and the approach is reviewed. Epidemiologic data suggest a decreased incidence of both cerebral hemorrhage and cerebral thrombosis over the last 10 years. Neurologic signs and symptoms include changes in mental status, motor function, sensation, vision and audition, and language. Laboratory studies and radiologic evaluation, including MRI or CT scan, will assist in differentiation of various stroke syndromes such as TIA, RIND, progressive stroke, intracerebral hemorrhage, and subarachnoid hemorrhage. The acute stroke management, medically and surgically, is reviewed along with the risks and complications that may occur following stroke.

DEFINITION OF STROKE

Stroke is the sudden onset of a neurologic deficit related to disruption of blood supply to an area of the brain. This may be a result of damage to the brain tissue from leaking of blood (hemorrhage) or from ischemic loss of brain tissue following an occlusion of a blood vessel from either a thrombus or an embolus. Stroke is common in the United States, currently ranking third among causes of death.

The evaluation of patients with a sudden onset of neurologic dysfunction has several goals. First, the diagnosis of stroke must be established. Other diagnoses that can mimic stroke include

---

E. Wayne Massey is Associate Professor of Neurology, Division of Neurology, Department of Medicine, Duke University Medical Center, Durham, NC 27710.

1

brain tumor, hydrocephalus, and metabolic, toxic and drug in-
duced encephalopathies. Once a diagnosis has been established,
the type of stroke syndrome should be defined in order to recommend appropriate therapy. A final goal of the evaluation is to
provide a documented record of function in order to determine if
progression has occurred. Thus, the full evaluation of the stroke
patient requires repeated examinations correlated with laboratory
and radiological evaluations.

EPIDEMIOLOGY

An explosive increase in epidemiologic studies of stroke has
generated considerable data over the last five years. The initial
step in evaluating epidemiologic studies is to make sure the diagnosis is correct. Different coding must be considered when comparing cerebrovascular disease codes from the eighth and ninth
ICD revisions (the International Classification of Diseases
adapted for use in the United States) (Table 1).

There does seem to be evidence for a decreasing incidence of
both cerebral hemorrhage and cerebral thrombosis, although how
long this decrease has been going on remains conjectural. This is
supported by the declining death rates which are recorded for
cerebrovascular disorders (Figure 1). Subarachnoid hemorrhage,
however, does not appear to share this decline. There does seem
to be a modest excess of males suffering all types of strokes, and
probably transient ischemic attacks (TIAs) as well. Age specific
rates in TIAs demonstrate much less of an increase with age than
in the case of cerebral thrombosis or hemorrhage.

Among whites, the prevalence rate for strokes is probably between 5 to 6 per 1000 population. The annual incidence rate is
between 1 and 2 per 1000. Death rate still seems to be about half
the incidence rate. All of these measures increase geometrically
with age, and by sex there is a modest male excess (3.1-1).

NEUROLOGICAL SIGNS AND SYMPTOMS

Stroke is characterized by its sudden onset and it may worsen
or regress after the initial onset. There are many signs and symp-

TABLE 1

CEREBROVASCULAR DISEASE (CVD) CODES ACCORDING TO
8TH (1968–1978) AND 9TH (1979–) REVISIONS OF
INTERNATIONAL CLASSIFICATION OF DISEASE

	8th Revision		9th Revision
Code	Title	Code	Title
430	subarachnoid hemorrhage	430	subarachnoid hemorrhage
431	cerebral hemorrhage	431	intracerebral hemorrhage
432	occlusion of precerebral arteries	432	other/specified intracranial hemorrhage
433	cerebral thrombosis	433	occlusion/stenosis of precerebral arteries
434	cerebral embolism	434	occlusion of cerebral arteries
435	transient cerebral ischemia	435	transient cerebral ischemia
436	acute but ill-defined CVD	436	acute but ill-defined CVD
437	generalized ischemic CVD	437	other and ill-defined CVD
438	other and ill-defined CVD	438	late effects of CVD

Figure 1. Annual age adjusted (US 1940) death rates per 100,000 population by sex and color, US 1915-1981. (From Kurtzke, 1985)

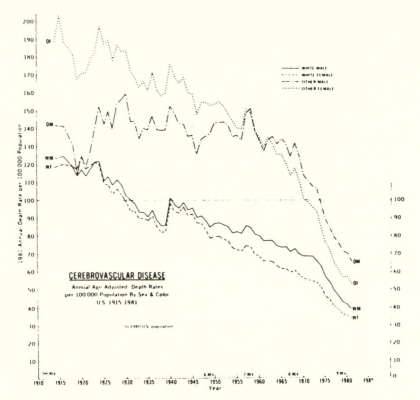

toms evaluated by the neurologist which will help to detect the location of the lesion and the subsequent progression of the illness.

The initial and subsequent neurological examinations should include all of the following categories:

1. Mental status. The initial evaluation is for orientation and memory as well as level of consciousness. Levels of consciousness include: (a) alert state, (b) lethargy, the patient may answer appropriately but will fall asleep when unattended, (c) obtundation, the patient may be aroused by verbal stimulation but otherwise is asleep, (d) stuporous, the patient requires physical stimulation to be aroused, and (e)

comatose, the patient does not respond to verbal or painful stimuli.

The evaluation of orientation and memory may be difficult in aphasic patients. The educational background of the patient and other environmental factors may inhibit the initial cognitive evaluation.

2. Motor function. Usually, patients with stroke present with a hemiparesis. Weakness may involve the arm, leg and face equally or one extremity greater than the other. Involvement of only one extremity is termed a monoparesis. Incoordination of the extremities or the trunk, termed ataxia, may be caused by involvement of cerebellar pathways or simply may be the result of muscle weakness. A patient is apraxic if he cannot initiate activities even when the motor deficit is not severe. Following a stroke the patient may have hypotonia or hypertonia; frequently, spasticity occurs.

3. Sensation. Sensory abnormalities of hypesthesia or anesthesia occur particularly in lesions of the parietal lobe. Clinicians should evaluate touch, vibration, position sense, pain, and temperature. It may also be helpful to test double simultaneous stimulation to evaluate for neglect of an extremity. Dysesthesias or actual pain on the side contralateral to the cerebral infarction may develop, particularly in the thalamic syndrome (Dejerine-Roussy syndrome).

4. Vision and Audition. Sudden loss of vision in one eye has been termed amaurosis fugax and is a result of transient occlusion of the branches of the retinal artery. When the cerebral cortex is involved, a hemianopsia, blindness in one side of the visual field, may occur. Diplopia, or double vision which occurs when two objects are perceived but only one object is present, develops in some stroke patients; this usually results from weakness of eye muscles following brainstem vascular insults affecting the eye control centers. Similarly, brainstem lesions may also produce vestibular or auditory dysfunction causing dizziness, light-headedness, or sudden loss of hearing in one ear.

5. Language. The disturbance of language function is termed aphasia. In right handed individuals, and in the majority of left handed persons as well, this most commonly occurs fol-

lowing left cerebral hemispheric damage. Aphasia may be (a) expressive (motor output difficulty) or (b) receptive (sensory input difficulty). Patients may have trouble with identifying objects or have inability to phonate or form words. Anomic aphasia is characterized by fluent speech and the ability to comprehend and repeat but difficulty in naming objects. In receptive aphasia, patients exhibit fluent speech but have difficulty comprehending spoken commands or repeating simple phrases. Confused patients may have difficulty understanding spoken words; this group of patients must be thoroughly evaluated.

6. Swallowing. Swallowing difficulty may occur with unilateral or bilateral neurologic involvement but it is more common with bilateral lesions and when brainstem areas are involved. Ability to swallow must be evaluated thoroughly in all patients with stroke and monitored to avoid subsequent aspiration of food material and possible pneumonia.

Findings of the neurological examination and a thorough knowledge of the distribution of the arterial blood supply to the brain assist the clinician in identifying the anatomic location of the lesion.

GENERAL PHYSICAL EXAMINATION

The physical examination must include measurement of vital signs since 20-25% of cerebral infarctions may be associated with cardiovascular disease. The presence of arrhythmias, bruits, hypertension, tachycardia, or abnormal ventilation may indicate an underlying cardiac dysfunction. A search for signs of metabolic disease or collagen vascular signs is important in some situations.

LABORATORY TESTS

Basic laboratory examination includes a complete blood count, urinalysis, serum electrolytes, blood glucose, blood urea nitrogen, and liver function tests. Elevated sedimentation rate is important in some patients (vasculitis). A sickle preparation is important in young black people with stroke, and hemoglobin and platelet abnormalities must be sought for in some individuals (i.e., thrombocytosis). Abnormalities in some of these blood tests may not be suspected from the physical examination. These tests are also useful to determine if the stroke is part of a systemic process involving other organs. Cardiac studies will include echocardiography, Holter monitor, and sometimes angiography. Pulmonary function tests are needed in some patients.

RADIOLOGIC EVALUATION

Computerized tomography (CT) frequently is obtained when a stroke patient is first seen. Computerized tomography is especially useful for detecting intracerebral or subarachnoid hemorrhage and for excluding other causes for acute neurological dysfunction. Computerized tomography evaluation often does not show an infarct in the first few days, thus cerebral infarctions are best seen by CT 5 to 7 days after a stroke. A CT scan indicates the size of infarction, the presence of brain swelling, and may detect hemorrhagic infarction.

Magnetic resonance imaging (MRI) may prove useful in classifying and following stroke patients. At present this form of imaging, however, does not seem helpful in evaluation of the acute stroke patient. More important, it is often difficult for a sick patient to lie still in the close confines of the scanner for the long period necessary to complete a study.

In selected patients, arteriography is used to visualize the cerebral circulation. Embolism often may be established with an arteriogram. Arteriography is useful in evaluating stroke patients with non-atherosclerotic disease, such as young patients without hypertension, diabetes, or a family history of cerebrovascular disease.

Cerebral blood flow studies are helpful in some cases. The Doppler or other noninvasive techniques to evaluate the carotid arteries frequently are useful.

E. Wayne Massey

STROKE SYNDROMES

The exact clinical classification of stroke is often difficult. For example, patients presenting with a hemiparesis and hemisensory loss may have damage in the contralateral internal capsule or in the brain stem. The internal capsule is supplied by a branch of the middle cerebral artery (the anterior circulation), while the brain stem is supplied by the basilar artery (the posterior circulation). It is difficult to differentiate between an intraparenchymal hemorrhage and a cerebral infarction without a CT scan. Additionally, clinicians are often uncertain as to whether a stroke results from thrombotic or embolic occlusion. A classification may be based on the neurological and physical examination, CT scan, and the subsequent clinical course (Table 2). This classification is useful in predicting prognosis and selecting appropriate management.

TABLE 2
STROKE SYNDROMES

— **TIA/RIND**
    Single
    Multiple
    Crescendo
— **Stroke in Evolution (Progressing)**
— **Completed Stroke (Ischemic infarction)**
    Embolic
    Thrombotic
    Lacunar
— **Intracerebral Hemorrhage (Parenchymal)**
— **Subarachnoid Hemorrhage**

TIA & RIND

Many stroke patients have a complete recovery. When the recovery takes place in less than 24 hours, the deficit is usually referred to as a *transient ischemic attack (TIA)*. When complete reversal occurs after 24 hours up to several months, the syndrome has been called a *reversible ischemic neurologic deficit (RIND)*. Although TIA originally was thought to represent a "pre-stroke" syndrome, as many as half of TIA patients have evidence of small cerebral infarcts, in an appropriate location for their symptoms, on CT scans. The exact mechanism underlying a TIA is not always clear. In some cases, symptoms may be caused by small platelet aggregates that temporarily lodge at branch points of small vessels, causing transient vascular occlusion. In others, symptoms result from transient inadequate perfusion of brain by collateral vessels because of pre-existing vascular stenosis or occlusion of the normal circulation. A dramatic example of this transitory circulatory insufficiency is the subclavian steal syndrome. Subclavian artery occlusion can be associated with cerebral symptoms when arm exercise steals blood from the cerebral circulation. This may be demonstrated by arteriography.

A RIND is often the clinical course of a first stroke. For example, in one study of stroke patients, 80% of those with first stroke had nearly complete recovery of neurological function, while recovery tended to be incomplete in patients suffering multiple strokes.

The appropriate management of patients with TIA or RIND is to evaluate and reduce their risk of a second stroke. The risk of a second stroke in patients with first stroke or TIA has been estimated at 8 to 10% per year for the subsequent two years. Surgical correction of severe carotid stenosis, daily aspirin, careful management of hypertension, weight reduction, exercise, and cessation of smoking are some commonly prescribed attempts to reduce this risk; however, scientific evidence that these approaches actually lower this risk is not concrete.

Progressing Stroke

Progressing stroke, or stroke-in-evolution, is present in roughly one-third of patients with thrombotic cerebral infarction and would probably be reported more often if patients arrived in the hospital soon after the onset of their symptoms.

Anticoagulation with heparin or coumadin is the most widely accepted therapy at present for progressing stroke. Agents designed to reduce cerebral edema, such as steroids and hyperosmolar agents, have generally not been of value in reducing morbidity or mortality or in enhancing recovery of function in patients with progressing stroke.

Several recent promising experimental approaches are being used. Hemodilution has been advocated to reduce blood viscosity and improve perfusion of ischemic brain areas. Hemodilution is attained by removing blood and replacing it with plasma expanders such as dextrans. Low molecular weight heparins (heparinoids) appear to have some of the antithrombotic properties of heparin without the anticoagulant properties and their use may prove of benefit in this type of stroke. Calcium channel antagonists could produce vascular dilatation and improve perfusion and these drugs are undergoing clinical trials.

Completed Stroke

Non-hemorrhagic acute neurological deficit almost always represents an *ischemic cerebral infarction*. The diagnosis of ischemic cerebral infarction is usually established when no other cause for neurological deficit is found. As already noted, CT examination often will not show infarction in the first few days although it is useful in excluding the possibility of intraparenchymal hemorrhage.

Once the diagnosis of cerebral infarction is established, attention should then be turned to determining if the infarction is due to embolic or to thrombotic occlusion of a cerebral vessel. This distinction is not always possible, but cerebral infarction from embolic occlusion represents 15 to 20% of all cerebral infarctions. The definite diagnosis of embolic occlusion rests on angiographic demonstration of emboli in the major cerebral arteries.

The importance of recognizing embolic occlusion stems from the 20 to 30% chance that the patient will suffer a second embolic episode. Most physicians recommend anticoagulation in patients with definite or probable embolic occlusion in the absence of either (1) CT evidence of a large cerebral infarction or (2) a hemorrhagic infarction of any size. Careful anticoagulation with adequate monitoring of anticoagulant activity is at present the best therapeutic approach to patients with proven or probable embolic disease.

Intracerebral Hemorrhage

The diagnosis of an *intracerebral hemorrhage* is best made with a computerized tomographic examination since even small collections of blood are easily detected by this means. The clinical presentation of intracerebral hemorrhage may be identical to that of cerebral infarction, but usually patients with hemorrhage have progressive signs and symptoms during the first 24 hours. It is important to carry out CT examination on every patient with a progressing stroke in whom anticoagulation is contemplated, since the presence of an intracerebral hemorrhage would be a contraindication for anticoagulation.

Surgical management of intracerebral hemorrhage is controversial. A prospective, randomized study of unselected patients comparing surgical and medical treatment is lacking. Surgeons frequently recommend removal of intracerebral hemorrhage in the non-dominant cerebral hemisphere when swelling and incipient brain herniation are present. Computerized tomography scans have detected small hemorrhages in many patients who would have been classified as cerebral infarction years ago. When all these patients with hemorrhage are considered, the prognosis is not as grave.

Subarachnoid Hemorrhage

Subarachnoid hemorrhage differs from other forms of stroke in its presentation. Depending on the severity and location of the bleeding, the clinical symptoms can vary from severe headache, mild confusion, and little neurological deficit to coma and death. The diagnosis of subarachnoid hemorrhage is made by demonstrating blood in the cerebrospinal fluid at the time of lumbar puncture. Computerized tomography examination will often detect subarachnoid blood, but rare cases have been described

where normal CT scans were found when subarachnoid hemorrhage was present. Therefore, evaluation of suspected subarachnoid hemorrhage requires a CT scan but a lumbar puncture
should be done when there is a strong suspicion.

Once the diagnosis of subarachnoid hemorrhage is made, it is
important to find the source of the bleeding. Although trauma,
aneurysm, and arteriovenous malformation are the usual causes
of subarachnoid hemorrhage, many cases are investigated without a cause revealed. When an aneurysm is identified with an
angiographic procedure, it is important to examine every cerebral
vessel because multiple aneurysms may be present.

A patient with subarachnoid hemorrhage from an aneurysm
stands at considerable risk of rebleeding. As a result, aneurysm
surgery is almost always recommended, but the timing of that
surgery depends on the clinical state of the patient. Alert patients
in good health come to early surgery, while comatose patients
with large amounts of subarachnoid blood make poor surgical
candidates. Surgery may be delayed until some recovery has
taken place, but early surgery is becoming more common even in
these cases.

A major complication of subarachnoid hemorrhage from any
of these conditions is arterial spasm. About 20% of patients have
the sudden onset of focal neurological dysfunction within a few
days of subarachnoid hemorrhage. Arteriography at that time
usually demonstrates narrowing of medium-sized arteries at several locations in the brain. The reason that these vessels undergo
spasm after exposure to blood in the cerebrospinal fluid is not
clear. In fact, the angiographic appearance of narrowed vessels
in spasm may not correlate with the anatomic location of the
focal deficit. Spasm is a major cause of death and disability in
patients with subarachnoid hemorrhage. No proven therapy exists at present, but raising the blood pressure appears helpful and
calcium channel blocking agents may be useful.

ACUTE STROKE MANAGEMENT

Approximately 20-25% of patients presenting to hospitals with
stroke die in the acute state. Many of these have an intraparenchymal cerebral hemorrhage or subarachnoid hemorrhage, but

occasional patients with cerebral infarction do not survive the acute stroke. In patients with cerebral infarction, the immediate danger comes from brain swelling in the area of infarction. The exact cause of cerebral edema in patients with infarction is not understood. Although a variety of medical therapies have been tried, including steroids, glycerol, and hyperventilation, none has been shown to be of benefit. Despite the lack of evidence to suggest that such therapies are valuable, when faced with a patient exhibiting brain swelling, one or more of these agents are usually employed.

MEDICAL MANAGEMENT

Acute Stroke

When the diagnosis of cerebral infarction is firmly established, it is important to observe the patient carefully. Ideally this is done in a hospital or emergency room for the first 24 to 48 hours. The major goal of this observation period is to detect any progression of symptoms. In addition, many patients have associated symptoms of cardiac disease or body fluid disturbance and careful attention to correction of these problems may ultimately improve outcome and prevent progression. Since one-third of stroke patients have progression of their neurological deficits after admission to the hospital, it is important to monitor vital signs and to perform frequent evaluations of motor strength, balance, speech, and level of consciousness in all patients immediately after a stroke. In addition, blood glucose levels should be monitored. Even if their deficits initially appear stable, progression can occur up to three to four days after the onset of stroke.

Blood Glucose

The admission blood glucose and the serum glucose level at the time of further stroke progression may be very important factors in the extent of cerebral infarction in any single patient. Although animal experiments have implicated glucose levels as an important determinant of stroke outcome, this has not been conclusively shown in humans. Early studies examining the relationship between blood glucose and stroke outcome in patients have differed in their results. Many stroke patients with high blood glucose on admission are diabetics and may have other causes of poor recovery. Regardless, these studies do indicate the possibility of some correlation between recovery from stroke and high admission blood glucose. At present, stroke care management should be planned on the assumption that an elevated blood glucose should be avoided particularly in the first 48 hours.

Anticoagulation

Anticoagulation with heparin is frequently used in (1) patients with progressing stroke, (2) cerebral infarction from probable or definite embolic origin, and (3) in patients with crescendo transient ischemic attacks. The efficacy of anticoagulation in these three clinical syndromes is debated but the evidence that anticoagulation prevents subsequent embolization seems the strongest. Whether anticoagulation actually improves function in progressive stroke or prevents stroke in patients with crescendo TIAs is unclear.

The major side effect of anticoagulation is minor bleeding, presenting as melena, hematuria, or hematemesis. Less common complications include massive hemorrhage into the retroperitoneal space or hemorrhage at the time of the lumbar puncture. Rare complications are heparin associated thrombocytopenia and intraparenchymal cerebral hemorrhage.

There is evidence that stroke patients with large infarctions are at risk of intraparenchymal hemorrhage from anticoagulation. In fact, the presence of a large cerebral infarct on CT scan is a contraindication to the use of anticoagulants. Successful management of stroke patients with anticoagulation requires careful control of their blood pressure and continued blood coagulation testing to allow adjustment of the anticoagulant drug dosage.

SURGICAL MANAGEMENT

Although several surgical procedures have been advocated in patients with acute stroke, none of them has proven beneficial. Patients who have had direct surgery on large extracranial blood vessels at the time of their cerebral infarction have generally not done well. In fact, this procedure is associated with a significantly high mortality and morbidity and is rarely performed. Extracranial-intracranial bypass was advocated for stroke patients with carotid obstructions, but a recent multi-national study showed no benefit to this surgical procedure.

Balloon angioplasty is carried out by passing a catheter into the stenotic or occluded artery and a thin guide wire is threaded across the stenosis or occlusion. A balloon in the tip of the catheter can be inflated to open the narrowed lining of the vessel. Angioplasty is used in coronary artery occlusive disease and myocardial infarction, but has not yet been successfully applied to cerebral infarction. It is likely that when the balloon is inflated, pieces of clot and plaque pass downstream in the blood vessel. In the heart, excellent collateral flow presumably prevents further myocardial damage from these microemboli. However, these microemboli produce neurological deficit when they pass downstream in cerebral vessels supplying the brain.

RISK FACTORS

There is much speculation about the cause of the decreasing incidence of stroke. Some experts feel that this reduced incidence has resulted from better attention to and treatment of high blood pressure and its sequelae. Careful management of hypertension is known to reduce the risk of stroke. Changes in nutrition and patterns of exercise in the 1970s and 1980s have led to decreased atherosclerosis. Whatever the cause of the decreased incidence of stroke, the fact that people are living longer in 1986 still makes stroke a major cause of neurological disability.

Heart disease. During the past decade, it has been recognized that stroke patients are at risk of heart attack. In fact, patients with stroke have the same risk of heart attack as patients with angina. Accordingly, stroke patients and their families should be advised to undertake changes in their lifestyles to prevent heart disease, such as low cholesterol diets, exercise, and instruction in cardiopulmonary resuscitation.

TIA/previous stroke. The risk of stroke is higher in patients with transient ischemic attacks or patients with previous stroke. This group of patients will benefit from careful examination for other risk factors such as hypertension, abnormal serum lipids, or unsuspected heart disease. These patients should adhere to proper diet, cease smoking, and take antihypertensive medication.

Patients with TIAs are usually evaluated for extracranial atherosclerotic disease of the carotid arteries with either ultrasound and similar noninvasive measures of carotid artery flow or with angiography. The presence of a stenotic carotid artery often leads to surgery. Carotid endarterectomy for carotid artery disease has become a common operation, but scientific studies of the ability of endarterectomy to prevent stroke are needed. Endarterectomy is being performed for indications ranging from a symptomatic carotid artery bruit to completed cerebral infarction. Many patients with reversible strokes and those with TIAs undergo carotid angiography and carotid surgery. A full evaluation of the procedure and its usefulness is desired.

Age. The risk of stroke increases with age. Current estimates are that 33% of Americans will be over the age of 65 by the year 2000. Thus even though the incidence of stroke is decreasing, stroke will likely continue to be a major source of disability and death.

Hypertension. High blood pressure has been recognized as a risk factor for stroke. Hypertension is associated with disease of small cerebral blood vessels that leads to small cerebral infarcts (lacunes) or intraparenchymal hemorrhages. Early hypertension is asymptomatic. Thus early detection depends on frequent blood pressure checks in normal people. If hypertension is detected, it should be controlled medically. There is substantial evidence that patients with moderate or severe hypertension can reduce their risk of stroke by taking appropriate antihypertensive medication. It is not so clear that patients with mild or labile hypertension benefit from antihypertensive medication, although it is usually prescribed.

Smoking. Since the risk of stroke is increased in cigarette smokers, individuals are well advised to avoid smoking.

Other factors. Hypercholesterolemia, obesity, and a familial tendency to stroke, although they have not been clearly proven, may also be risk factors.

COMPLICATIONS OF STROKE

Cerebral edema. The most serious complication of stroke is cerebral edema with swelling of the cerebral hemisphere, leading eventually to herniation of the brain and death. As previously discussed, this is probably the most common cause of mortality in acute cerebral infarction. Cerebral edema can be detected by CT scan and usually begins 48-72 hours after cerebral infarction. Thus, patients may present with a neurological deficit which appears stable for the first 24-48 hours and then progress, with alteration in consciousness and worsening of the initial deficit due to cerebral edema. A CT scan may show swelling of the infarcted hemisphere with incipient herniation.

Intraparenchymal hemorrhage. Hemorrhage into a cerebral infarction can be a complication of stroke in anticoagulated patients. This type of intraparenchymal hemorrhage is different from the hemorrhagic cerebral infarction seen in stroke patients with embolic occlusions and can sometimes be determined from the pattern on CT scan. Either type of hemorrhage can produce cerebral edema and hemisphere swelling and represents a serious complication of stroke.

Recurrent stroke. As mentioned earlier, first strokes often are reversible. By contrast, second or multiple strokes have a more serious prognosis. Thus, recurrent stroke is a serious complication of stroke and can best be prevented by attempting to reduce risk factors. In patients with stroke from embolic causes, recurrent stroke can be prevented by anticoagulation for several months when the risk of a new embolization appears the greatest.

Aspiration pneumonia. Many patients with hemispheric and brain stem cerebral infarction will have trouble swallowing liquids, placing them in danger of aspirating fluids or secretions into their lungs. Aspiration commonly leads to pulmonary infection. Swallowing evaluation, including video fluoroscopy, should be used frequently.

Deep vein thrombosis. Any time a patient is immobilized, the possibility of deep vein thrombosis (DVT) in an extremity is present. This risk is greatest in stroke patients with muscle weakness or paralysis because of diminished venous blood flow in the affected extremity. The presence of congestive heart failure and paralysis is a particularly dangerous combination. A major concern in deep vein thrombosis is that clot may break loose and pass upstream to lodge in the lung. Pulmonary embolism is frequently fatal.

Decubitus ulcer. Adequate skin care is important in the paralyzed stroke patient. Pressure on skin over boney prominences reduces blood flow and leads to skin breakdown, ulceration, and infection. Decubitus ulcers can be difficult to treat, at times requiring intensive nursing management (frequent turning, application of antiseptic solutions, antibiotics). Sepsis from decubitus ulcers can cause death.

Falls. Motor deficits place stroke patients at risk of episodes of imbalance during normal activity, that can lead to falls. Resultant head injury, bone fractures, and other disabilities can be life-threatening. It is important for patients with stroke to learn to avoid situations where their balance or motor strength may be impaired and where the danger of falling can lead to serious complications.

Dysphagia. Difficulty in swallowing solids can occur in stroke patients and can be permanent. In these patients, gastrostomy may be necessary for administering food and liquids directly into the stomach, often requiring intensive nursing care. Silent aspiration may be frequent.

Dementia. Cerebral infarction is associated with several clinical syndromes of dementia. Patients with multiple cerebral infarctions, especially when both cerebral hemispheres are involved, may develop problems with memory, comprehension, and cognition. Hypertensive individuals may have small multiple cerebral infarctions which are not apparent as a stroke. These patients may come to medical attention with a multi-infarct dementia (M.I.D.) mimicking senile dementia of the Alzheimer's type. Small cerebral infarcts of the subcortical white matter have been recognized as a common cause of dementia and called subcortical arteriosclerotic encephalopathy (Binswanger's disease).

Many patients with Binswanger's disease present with a dementing illness and most have underlying hypertension.

Depression. Cerebral infarction may be associated with psychiatric depression. In some cases, the emotional disorder is a reaction to the suddenly acquired handicap resulting from stroke. In other cases, there appears to be a biological relationship between the infarction and subsequent depression. Some evidence suggests that specific infarction of the left frontal lobe is associated with depression, suggesting a direct effect.

FUTURE MANAGEMENT

The greatest advances in management of stroke are likely to result from a greater appreciation of the importance of treating patients immediately after the beginning of their symptoms. It is possible that rapid attention to blood viscosity and oxygenation within the first few minutes of infarction may be of great benefit. The practical problem of getting medical attention to patients as soon as possible probably will not be addressed until medical treatments become available and are proven of value in the immediate period after stroke.

A collection of drugs for the treatment of the patient with cerebral infarction is starting to emerge. Agents may become available that will enhance the recovery of function. Just as there are agents which may promote recovery of function, it is likely that some drugs may actually worsen recovery after stroke and should be avoided. Since many of these patients have heart disease, hypertension, diabetes, and complications of stroke, it is not surprising that stroke patients often receive a variety of medications during the period following their stroke. The future may allow a more rational approach to the drugs prescribed.

REFERENCES

Basmajian JV, Kirby RL: Medical Rehabilitation. Baltimore, Williams & Wilkins, 1984

Kurland LT, Kurtzke JF: Epidemiology of Neurologic and Sense Organ Disorders. Cambridge, Harvard Univ Press, 1973

Kurtzke J: Epidemiology of cerebrovascular disease, in *Cerebrovascular Survey Report for the National Institute of Neurological and Communicative Disorders and Stroke*. McDowell F, Chaplan L (eds), Revised 1985 pp 1-34

Mohr JP et al: Harvard Cooperative Stroke Registry: a prospective Registry. Neurology 28: 754-762, 1978

Moore JC: Neuroanatomical considerations relating to recovery of function following brain lesions. In Recovery of Functions: Theoretical Consideration for Brain Injury Rehabilitation; edited by Bach-y-Rita P. Baltimore, University Park Press, 1980

Toole JF: Cerebrovascular Disorders. 3rd Edition, New York, Raven Press, 1984

Stroke: Characteristics of the Central Nervous System that Influence Its Clinical Expression

Eleanor F. Branch, PhD, PT

SUMMARY. This paper addresses certain anatomic and hemo-dynamic characteristics of the central nervous system that may modify the pathological and clinical features of stroke. Illustrated case studies emphasize common clinical situations in which stroke occurs; the repair process in the brain following infarction; the effects of brain herniation; and the significance of anasto-motic channels and collateral circulation in protecting the brain from ischemic injury.

Cerebral ischemia accounts for the vast majority of stroke syndromes. The morphologic expression and extent of an infarction, as well as its clinical presentation, however, may be modified by several anatomic and hemodynamic features of the central nervous system.[1] Knowledge of these features enables one to (1) understand and appreciate better the variability of signs and symptoms with which stroke patients present, even in situations in which identical arteries may be occluded by a thrombus or an embolus; and (2) be more cognizant of how extensive the residual loss of brain tissue may be in patients who survive cerebro-

Dr. Branch is an associate professor and Director of Graduate Studies in the Department of Physical Therapy, Duke University Medical Center, Durham, NC 27710.

The author wishes to acknowledge the Department of Pathology, Duke University Medical Center, for allowing her access to its photography collection, and to thank Mrs. Nancy Marshburn for her artistic assistance in the preparation of this article.

vascular accidents. This article will review some of these modi-
fying features and present clinical examples of their impact upon
the outcome of cerebral ischemia.

ANATOMIC FEATURES

Repair Following Ischemia

Neurons are classified as permanent cells, so that destruction
of a neuron, whether it is in the central nervous system or in one
of the ganglia, represents a permanent loss. Repair of neural tissue in response to ischemia, therefore, cannot occur as the result
of neuronal replication. Instead, the repair process following
neuronal death involves a proliferative response by a type of cell
called the astrocyte, indigenous to the central nervous system.
Although there are important differences between the two cell
types, astrocytes may be considered the central nervous system
analogue of the fibroblast, a cell responsible for collagenous scar
formation in other areas of the body; except for a few fibroblasts
in the walls of larger blood vessels and in the meninges, these
cells do not exist in the central nervous system.

Cerebral artery occlusion of sufficient duration produces tissue
death and necrosis, in which the brain undergoes a series of sequential anatomic changes that are similar no matter the location
of the damaged area.[2] During the first 12 to 24 hours, usually no
visible gross alterations can be demonstrated, although the neural
tissue is already irreparably damaged. By 24 to 36 hours, the
damaged zone appears pale and soft, and the demarcation between the white and grey matter becomes indistinct. Swelling is
apparent and sometimes accompanied by a certain degree of vascular congestion, imparting a duskiness to the tissue. From 2 to
10 days, the boundaries of the infarcted area gradually become
better defined as swelling decreases. After 10 days, a process of
liquefaction begins, and from the third to fourth week onward
cavitation becomes increasingly more evident. Cavitation is a reflection of the fact that the dead tissue is being removed by mac-
rophages,[2] and the astrocytes, which have proliferated and hypertrophied, are forming a "glial scar" around the periphery of the
lesion. It is the intertwining of astrocyte cell processes that cre-
ates this "scar." The final cystic cavity frequently has ragged

outlines and may be intersected by vascular connective tissue strands; in the case of a large infarct, 10 or more years may be required for this stage to be reached.[3] Unlike early expansile lesions, old infarcts retract and permit expansion of an adjacent ventricle. This repair process is quite different from that seen in other areas of the body, such as the skin, where fibroblasts lay down a firm collagenous scar.

The Encasement of the Brain by the Skull

The rigid encasement of the brain by the skull provides great protection against injury, at the same time becoming detrimental when there is an expansion of the intracranial contents. Such expansion may occur because of the edema associated with cerebral ischemia, following brain trauma, and when there are space-occupying lesions, such as tumors, in the central nervous system. In the adult, the rigid bony skull limits expansion of the brain volume, and mounting intracranial pressure results. The effects of raised intracranial pressure depend on the rate of the increasing pressure and include (1) headache, (2) vomiting, (3) impaired consciousness, (4) bulging of the optic disc (papilledema), with engorgement of its vessels, (5) rising systemic blood pressure and reflex slowing of the pulse, and (6) herniation of the brain.

Herniation is the name given to displacement of part of the brain from one dural compartment to another and is a potentially serious consequence of raised intracranial pressure.[1] The effects of herniation depend on the direction of displacement (Figure 1). In unilateral lesions of the frontal or parietal lobes, herniation of the cingulate gyrus can occur beneath the free edge of the falx cerebri; this type of herniation may lead to compression of the anterior cerebral arteries against the falx, and secondary brain infarction. Expanding masses above the tentorium cerebelli — the dural shelf separating the cerebellum from the occipital lobes — can cause displacement of the uncus of the temporal lobe medially over the free edge of the tentorium. This may result in compression of the ipsilateral, or in some cases contralateral, cerebral peduncle and corticospinal tract, and clinical signs of hemiparesis and hyperreflexia; compression of the third nerve, leading to homolateral pupil dilatation, ptosis, and third nerve palsy; and shift of the brain stem caudally, resulting ultimately in hemor-

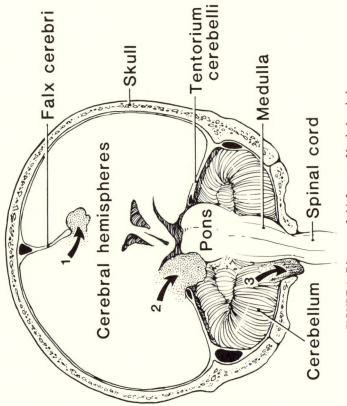

Falx cerebri

Skull

Tentorium cerebelli

Medulla

Spinal cord

Cerebellum

Pons

Cerebral hemispheres

FIGURE 1. Diagram of chief types of brain herniation.
1. Cingulate gyrus (falx) herniation
2. Temporal lobe (tentorial) herniation
3. Cerebellar (foramen magnum) herniation

rhages in the midbrain and pons, and death. Such tentorial herniation also may be associated with compression of the posterior cerebral artery (PCA) as it courses around the peduncle on its way to the occipital lobe; infarction of part of the visual cortex also may occur, with resultant contralateral homonymous hemianopsia.[2] An overall increase in pressure within the cranium from a lesion in the posterior fossa can cause herniation of the cerebellum through the foramen magnum, leading to compression of the medulla and usually resulting in immediate death. Cerebral ischemia resulting in stroke may be associated with sufficient edema of the brain to cause herniation, and may be life threatening in the case of large infarctions because of the described potential for producing brain stem compression and death.

Correlation Between Function and Location

Unlike some organs such as the liver, where one liver parenchymal cell is much like another and functions in a similar way, the clinical effect of a lesion in the central nervous system depends largely on its location. Contralateral hemiparesis may be produced following ischemic necrosis in the precentral gyrus of the frontal cortex; the same degree of necrosis in the superior temporal gyrus causes a receptive aphasia. In addition, the size of the lesion may be particularly significant. A small infarction of the prefrontal cortex may not produce symptoms for the patient; in contrast, a lesion of the same size in the medulla may cause instant death. This correlation between function and location in the nervous system is of great value to the clinician. Certain signs or symptoms may enable the examiner to infer the exact location of the causative lesion.

HEMODYNAMIC FEATURES

The extent of brain infarction, following occlusion of an arterial vessel by a thrombus or an embolus, is influenced by several hemodynamic factors; that is, not all occlusions will result in tissue death and in clinical signs and symptoms.[1] Anastomotic channels exist between cortical branches of the anterior, middle, and posterior cerebral arteries over the surface of the cerebral cortex; between the external carotid and ophthalmic arteries in the orbit; between the vertebral and basilar arteries over the surface of the cerebellum; and between the posterior (vertebrobasilar) and the anterior (carotid) circulation via the circle of Willis at the base of the brain (Figure 2). These rich anastomotic networks help to protect the brain by allowing for alternate routes which can circumvent obstruction in any of the main arteries supplying the brain. For example, thrombosis of the anterior cerebral artery (ACA) just distal to its origin from the internal carotid artery might not result in appreciable damage to the cortex fed by that artery because of blood flowing from the opposite ACA, through the anterior communicating artery (Figure 3); cortical anastomoses might be of some benefit as well. In occlusion of the basilar artery, circulation may be maintained by flow from the internal carotid arteries via the circle of Willis and by anastomotic channels between the posterior inferior cerebellar and the superior cerebellar arteries (Figure 3).[4]

In spite of these prevalent anastomotic connections, such vascular arrangements may vary from individual to individual (Case I),[2] and the channels themselves may be occluded by atherosclerosis and, therefore, be ineffective in preventing tissue damage. In addition, in a substantial number of cerebral infarcts, examination of the arterial tree fails to reveal structural occlusion (Case II).[1,5] The etiology of such infarcts has been attributed to factors such as arterial "spasm," emboli which have undergone lysis, and hypoperfusion coincident with a hypotensive episode.[6]

A thrombus that leads to gradual occlusion of a vessel frequently will facilitate the development of anastomotic channels and the patient may be asymptomatic (at least until an additional compromise of circulation occurs, as in Case III). An embolus, on the other hand, produces sudden occlusion. For these reasons, infarction resulting from thrombosis may be more limited in extent than that produced by an embolus.[5] If the embolus is lysed rapidly, however, blood flow may be reestablished and extensive damage may be prevented.

CASE STUDIES

The following case studies will serve to illustrate common clinical situations in which cerebrovascular accidents may occur,

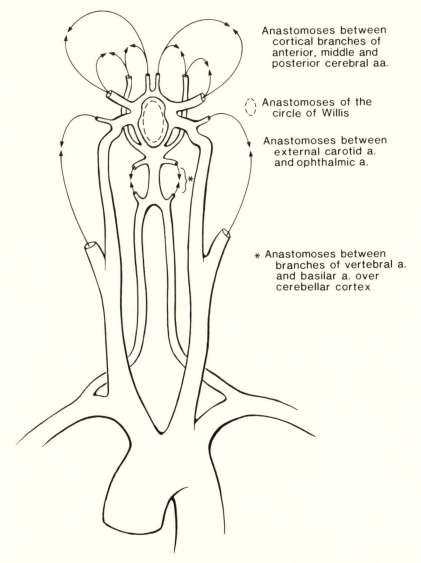

FIGURE 2. Diagram of the carotid and vertebrobasilar circulations and their chief anastomotic channels. (Adapted from Escourolle, R., Poirier, J. & Rubinstein, L. J. (trans) (1978): *Manual of Basic Neuropathology*, 2nd ed.; Philadelphia: W. B. Saunders; reprinted from *Stroke Rehabilitation: Recovery of Motor Control*, ed. Duncan & Badke, 1987, p54, with permission of Year Book Medical Publishers.)

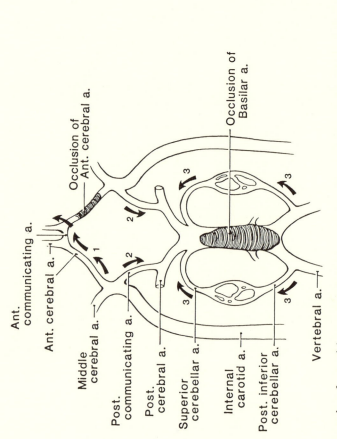

Ant.
communicating a.

Ant. cerebral a.

Middle
cerebral a.

Post.
communicating a.

Post.
cerebral a.

Superior
cerebellar a.

Internal
carotid a.

Post. inferior
cerebellar a.

Vertebral a.

Occlusion of
Ant. cerebral a.

Occlusion of
Basilar a.

FIGURE 3. Diagram of examples of potential routes to circumvent cerebral artery obstruction. (Adapted from Fields, W. S. (1974). Aortocranial occlusive vascular disease (stroke). *Clinical Symposia.* Summit, NJ: CIBA Pharmaceutical Co., Vol. 26, Number 4.) In occlusion of one ACA, just distal to its origin, flow may be maintained from the opposite ACA through the anterior communicating artery-1. In a proximal occlusion of the basilar artery, the internal carotid arteries may supply the posterior circulation via the posterior communicating arteries-2; in addition, blood flow between branches of the vertebral and basilar arteries may provide bypass channels-3.

as well as some of the anatomic and hemodynamic features of the nervous system which we have been discussing.

Case I

This 67 year old white man, with a history of adult onset diabetes mellitus, hypertension, and congestive heart failure, temporarily lost vision in his right eye (i.e., a transient ischemic attack) one month prior to admission to the hospital; three weeks later, the patient noted bilateral blurred vision, which also cleared. One day prior to admission, the patient observed that, while watching television, he saw only one side of the screen. In the hospital, neurological evaluation revealed a left homonymous hemianopsia, and a computerized tomography (CT) scan demonstrated a large area of infarction in the right occipital lobe. On the fifth hospital day, the patient was found without pulse and other vital signs; the cause of death was attributed to heart failure.

At autopsy, the right occipital lobe was soft and necrotic, with early cystic changes compatible with a two-week-old infarction (Figure 4). Examination of the circle of Willis revealed an anomaly (Figure 5). The left posterior communicating artery was of large (embryonic) caliber and supplied the left PCA from the internal carotid system; no direct connection with the basilar artery was present. On the right, the basilar artery was the sole source of blood supply to the right PCA (and thus to the right occipital lobe) because the right posterior communicating artery was vestigial. A thrombus was present in the right PCA four centimeters from its origin. All the major cerebral vessels showed severe atherosclerosis.

This case illustrates

1. a common anatomic variation of the circle of Willis and its branches.[2] In this setting of severe atherosclerosis and thrombotic occlusion of the right PCA, a variation which usually would be functionally insignificant might well have compromised the potential for collateral blood flow to the occipital lobe.
2. the gross features of a cerebral infarct of approximately two weeks' duration.

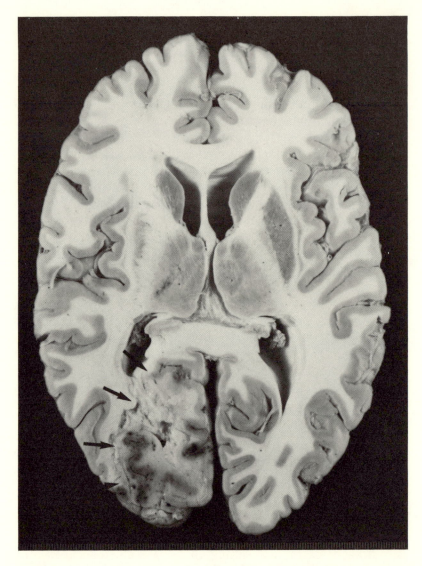

FIGURE 4. (Case I) Horizontal section of the brain, viewed from below, showing a cerebral infarct of approximately two weeks' duration, in the distribution of the right PCA (arrows).

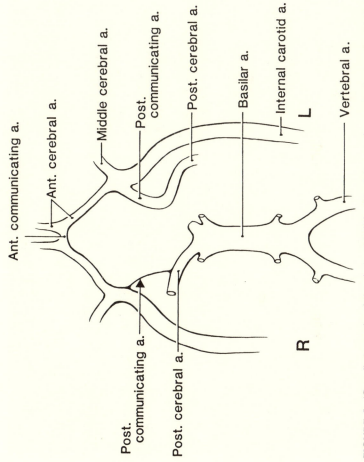

FIGURE 5. (Case I) Anomaly of the circle of Willis. The left posterior cerebral artery is supplied exclusively from the internal carotid system. The right posterior cerebral artery receives flow solely from the vertebrobasilar system.

31

Case II

This 62 year old white woman, with a five year history of atrial fibrillation and increasing signs of congestive heart failure, was brought to the Emergency Room because she exhibited garbled speech. Approximately one week later, the patient developed expressive aphasia, obtundation, decerebrate posturing, and fixed pupils. She expired a day later.

At autopsy, there was softening of the brain in the distribution of the left middle cerebral artery (MCA), with relative sparing of the basal ganglia; occlusion of the left lateral ventricle by swelling; and herniation of the left cingulate gyrus (Figure 6A) and temporal lobe (Figure 6B). No appreciable atherosclerosis of the cerebral blood vessels and no evidence of occlusion by thrombi or emboli were noted.

This case illustrates

1. significant cerebral infarction in the absence of any apparent structural occlusion in the cerebral vasculature. In this patient, the brain lesion was attributed to hypoperfusion of the brain associated with failing cardiac function.
2. the gross features of a cerebral infarct compatible with an ischemic event occurring 2 to 10 days earlier.
3. herniation of the brain resulting from increased intracranial pressure associated with cerebral edema.

Case III

A 45 year old white woman, with a history of angina, myocardial infarction, and hypertension, experienced a right hemiparesis, decreased sensation in the right upper extremity, aphasia, and altered mental status, during a cardiac catherization. A CT scan six days later demonstrated infarctions in the distribution of the left MCA and the left PCA, as well as evidence of cerebral edema; the same day, the patient developed a dilated left pupil. Eight days later, the patient became comatose, exhibited bilateral fixed and dilated pupils, suffered a cardiac arrest, and expired — 14 days following the catherization. The patient was believed to have died of cerebral edema, and from bleeding of gastrointesti-

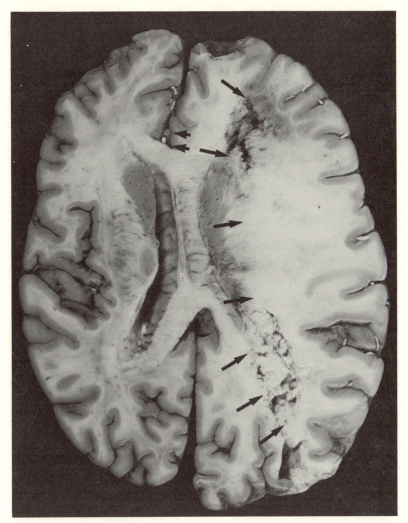

FIGURE 6A. (Case II) Horizontal section of the brain, viewed from below, showing a cerebral infarct in the distribution of the left MCA (long arrows). Note that the left lateral ventricle is occluded by marked swelling of the left cerebral hemisphere, and that there is herniation of the left cingulate gyrus (short arrows).

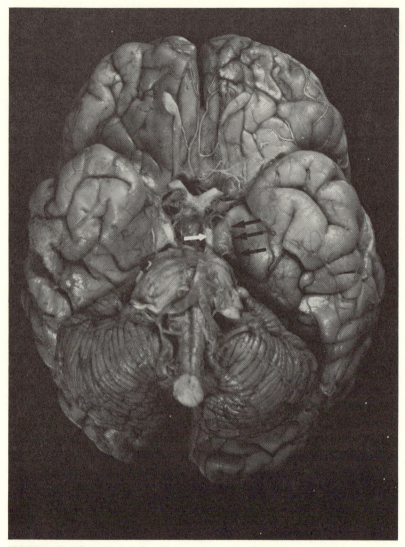

FIGURE 6B. (Case II) Inferior view of the brain. The marked swelling of the left cerebral hemisphere has displaced the temporal lobe over free edge of the tentorium, with resultant grooving of the uncus (black arrows) and pressure on the third nerve (white arrow).

nal ulcers which could have resulted from steroids used to treat the edema.

At autopsy, the left cerebral hemisphere was soft and swollen, and grossly the infarctions in the distribution of the left MCA and PCA were relatively well demarcated and consistent with an ischemic event at the time of the catherization two weeks earlier (Figure 7). There was minimal atherosclerosis of the vessels of the circle of Willis. The right common carotid artery, however, showed marked atherosclerotic changes and was totally occluded by an old, well-organized thrombus; 75% stenosis of the origin of the left vertebral artery was evident. The left common carotid artery was stenotic at its origin, which was blocked by a cholesterol embolus; a fresh thrombus associated with the embolus filled the artery over a 3 centimeter length.

This case illustrates

1. a patient, with a long standing history of total occlusion of the right common carotid artery and narrowing of the left common carotid and the left vertebral arteries, who did not exhibit neurological impairment until an additional compromise of the cerebral circulation (the cholesterol embolus released during the catherization) occurred. It only may be speculated that preservation of the blood flow to the left anterior cerebral artery was a result of collateral blood flow through the vertebrobasilar system and the circle of Willis (Figure 2).
2. the gross features of a cerebral infarct of approximately two weeks' duration.

Case IV

A 42 year old black man, with a history of high blood pressure, myocardial infarction, and two-vessel coronary artery bypass surgery, suddenly developed a right hemiplegia, four months following the surgery. Cardiac studies revealed a thrombus attached to the lining of the left ventricle (i.e., a mural thrombus); this thrombus was thought to have embolized to the cerebrum. A CT scan revealed a large infarction in the distribu-

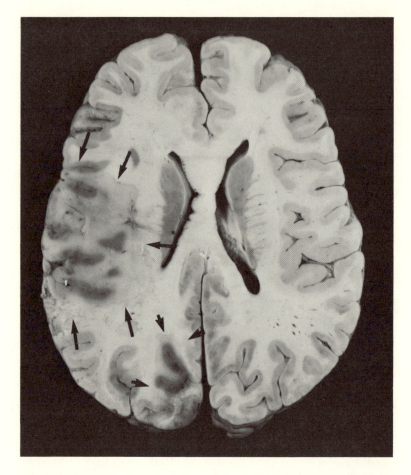

FIGURE 7. (Case III) Horizontal section of the brain, viewed from above, showing cerebral infarcts of approximately two weeks' duration. The area of infarction in the distribution of the left MCA (long arrows) is somewhat better defined than that in the distribution of the left PCA (short arrows). The left hemisphere appears swollen.

tion of the left MCA, as well as evidence of herniation. The patient developed aspiration pneumonia, and died approximately one month after the neurological event.

Autopsy revealed a large area of softening and beginning liquefaction of tissue in the distribution of the left MCA (Figure 8), and a thromboembolus filled the lumen of that artery distal to the branches to the basal ganglia. Slight herniation of the cingulate

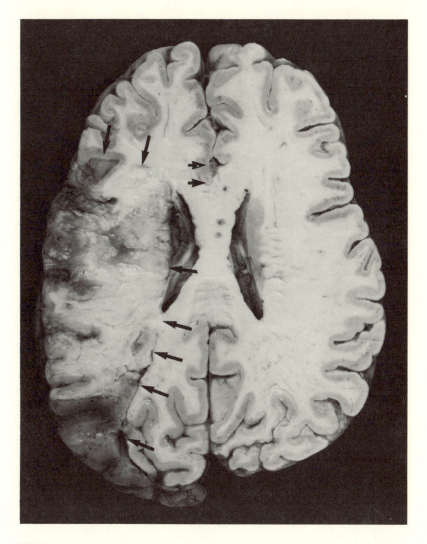

FIGURE 8. (Case IV) Horizontal section of the brain, viewed from above, showing a cerebral infarct of approximately one month's duration. Note large area of softening in the distribution of the left MCA (long arrows) and slight herniation of the left cingulate gyrus (short arrows). This infarct shows early liquefactive changes.

gyrus under the falx, from left to right, was seen, and grooving of the left uncus denoted transtentorial herniation.

This case illustrates

1. an example of cerebral embolization from a mural thrombus in the heart, overlying a myocardial infarction;[1,2,5] as most commonly occurs in such situations, the embolus traveled into the carotid circulation[2,6] to terminate in the MCA.
2. the gross features of a cerebral infarct of approximately one month's duration.

Case V

A 30 year old retarded white man, with a left hemiplegia and seizures from birth, suffered extensive thermal burns. Two weeks later, the patient died of sepsis and kidney failure. At autopsy, the right side of the skull was decreased in size and the right cerebral cortex was atrophic and cystic, in the distribution of the MCA (Figure 9A). The cyst extended from the pia to the basal ganglia, and the right internal capsule was markedly atrophic (Fig. 9B).

This case illustrates,

1. the gross features of cerebral infarction of 30 years' duration, and the extensive residual loss of cerebral tissue that may be seen in patients surviving cerebrovascular accidents.
2. the atrophy and loss of fibers (in the internal capsule) whose neuronal cell bodies were destroyed by ischemic injury at birth.

Case VI

This 62 year old white woman was brought to the emergency room, from a nursing home, with complaints of abdominal pain. She had experienced an extensive right hemisphere stroke four years earlier, and also had a history of angina, hypertension, congestive heart failure, aorto-femoral bypass graft surgery for occlusive peripheral arterial disease, and carotid endarterectomy. Gall bladder surgery was performed two days following admis-

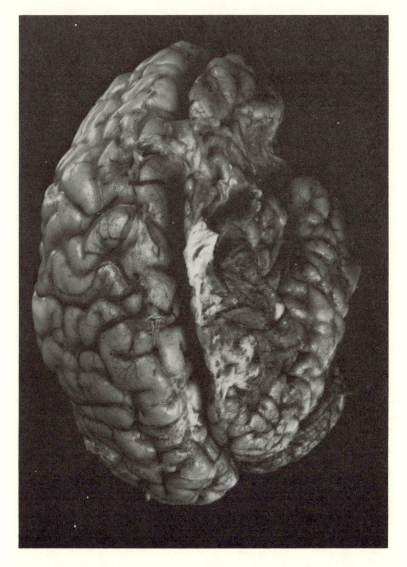

FIGURE 9A. (Case V) Superior view of the brain showing an infarction of 30 years' duration, with extensive loss of cerebral tissue in the distribution of the right MCA.

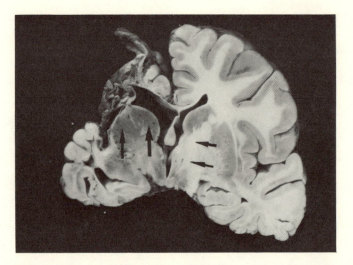

FIGURE 9B. (Case V) Frontal section of the brain in Figure 9A. The cyst extends from the meninges to the right basal ganglia (long arrows), which have a mottled appearance when compared to the left side. Note the normal configuration of the left internal capsule (short arrows) and the atrophy of this tract on the right side.

sion to the hospital, and the second day postoperatively the patient's mental status deteriorated. She experienced an acute myocardial infarction and died on the fourth postoperative day.

At autopsy, there was marked cyst formation in the brain in the distribution of the right MCA, with retraction of the meninges and dilation of the right lateral ventricle (Figure 10). The cyst reached from the cerebral cortex to include parts of the basal ganglia and the posterior limb of the internal capsule, with marked atrophy of the ipsilateral cerebral peduncle. The thalamus and the head of the caudate nucleus (supplied by other cerebral arteries) were spared.

This case illustrates

1. the gross features of cerebral infarction occurring four years earlier: cyst formation, retraction of tissue, and dilation of the adjacent ventricle. This is in sharp contrast to early expansile lesions (Case II & Case III).
2. the common association of atherosclerotic coronary artery, cerebral artery, and peripheral artery disease.

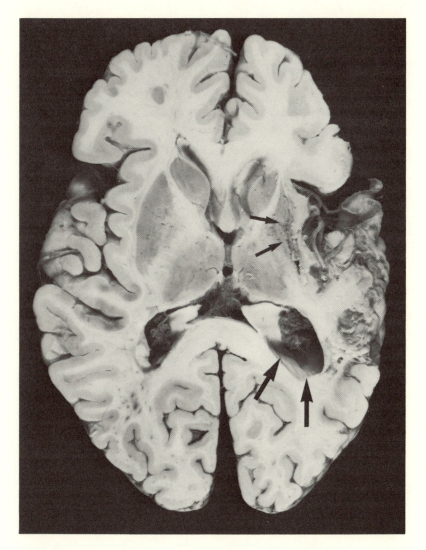

FIGURE 10. (Case VI) Horizontal section of the brain, viewed from above, showing an infarct of four years' duration, in the right MCA distribution. Dilation of the right lateral ventricle (large arrows) reflects the retraction (rather than swelling) characteristic of old infarctions (compare to Figure 6A, Case II). The cyst includes part of the right basal ganglia and internal capsule (small arrows).

NOTES

1. Escourolle R, Poirier J., Rubinstein LJ (trans.): Manual of Basic Neuropathology, ed 2. Philadelphia, WB Saunders Company, 1978

2. Burger PC, Vogel FS: Cerebrovascular Disease. Teaching Monograph Series published in The American Journal of Pathology, Bethesda, Maryland, The American Association of Pathologists, 1978

3. Weller RO: Color Atlas of Neuropathology. New York, Oxford University Press, 1984

4. Fields WS: Aortocranial Occlusive Vascular Disease (Stroke). Clinical Symposia. Summit, NJ, CIBA Pharmaceutical Company, Vol 26, Number 4, 1974

5. An ad hoc committee established by the Advisory Council for the National Institute of Neurological Diseases and Blindness, Public Health Service: A Classification and Outline of Cerebrovascular Diseases. Reprinted from Neurology 8: May, 1958

6. Toole JF: Cerebrovascular Disorders, ed 3. New York, Raven Press, 1984

Weakness in the
Stroke Patient:
A Review

Richard W. Bohannon, MS, PT

SUMMARY. As a controversy exists regarding weakness and its measurement in hemiplegic stroke patients, this review was written. In keeping with a proposed operational definition of weakness, I provide a perspective supportive of strength measurement in stroke patients. The weakness, which is a function of such factors as lesion location, motor unit recruitment, muscle changes and antagonist restraint, does improve following stroke. This improvement is discussed, as is the relationship between strength and function.

Predominantly unilateral weakness (hemiplegia) is by far the most frequently noted sequela of cerebrovascular accidents (CVAs).[1] Whether stroke patients are truly weak and whether strength measurement is valuable in these patients are topics of some controversy. The purpose of this review is to address such controversy. To achieve my purpose, I will (1) propose an operational definition of weakness that can be applied to stroke patients; (2) discuss the measurement of strength in stroke patients and the findings of studies in which strength has been measured; and (3) describe some of the factors underlying the strength deficits demonstrated by these patients. Finally, the recovery of strength and its relationship to function will be addressed.

Mr. Bohannon is Chief, Department of Physical Therapy, Southeastern Regional Rehabilitation Center, Cape Fear Valley Medical Center, P. O. Box 2000, Fayetteville, NC 28302.

WEAKNESS DEFINED

Problems with the use of terms "strength" and "weakness," notwithstanding, I will use them in this review in lieu of other vague terms such as "muscle performance."[2] This choice of terms follows a desire to exclude from the text any extensive discussion of motor control or coordination,[3] which might be subsumed under a concept such as muscle performance. If the scope of this discussion is to be limited, the issue of motor control must be largely avoided, even if it is potentially related to strength and of proven importance to functional performance in stroke patients.[4]

Any definition of weakness, of course, is inexorably tied to that of strength. In this paper, strength is defined as the capacity of a muscle or a group of muscles to bring force to bear on the environment. The ramifications of this force can be the maintenance of joint and body positions against external forces or the movement of one or more joints in space against varying counterforces. For my purpose weakness is defined as any deficit of "normal" strength. The greater the deficit the greater the weakness, whether the deficit is relative to a patient's premorbid status or some population norm.

STRENGTH MEASUREMENT

Although the measurement of strength is a fundamental part of the physical therapy assessment of patients with many disorders, a number of respected authors have questioned the validity of strength measurements in patients with central nervous system lesions. In their text on muscle testing, Daniels and Worthingham express concern over the possible influence of tone and synergies during attempts to test the strength of patients with brain lesions.[5] Bobath claims that the testing of muscles of stroke patients is "unreliable" because of the opposition of spastic or co-contracting antagonists, the presence of sensory deficits, the tendency of muscles to work in mass patterns, and the absence of synergistic fixation during testing.[6] She claims, furthermore, that limitations in joint range and weakness are secondary to problems of coordination in posture and movement. Davies expresses a similar belief, stating that, in the presence of antagonist spasticity, the accurate estimation of agonist force is impossible.[7] She cites the example of ankle dorsiflexion in the presence of hypertonus of the calf muscles. Perhaps concerns such as these underlie Chan's recommendation that the degree of paralysis or paresis be estimated by observation of a patient's tendency to limb synergies and ability to break or move out of synergy.[8]

The aforementioned perspectives notwithstanding, numerous investigations have been conducted in which traditional ordinal grading schemes or instruments have been used to measure the strength of hemiplegic stroke patients. Published ordinal measuring schemes use scales of three to six categories. McDowell and Louis used a three-category scale (complete paralysis, paresis, no weakness).[9] Bard and Hirschberg, who qualified that their scale measured motion which should not be confused with strength or function, used a four-point scale.[10] They graded movement as zero (none), trace (less than one-quarter range), partial (one-quarter to three-quarter range), and full (greater than three-quarter range). Demeurisse and associates[11] and Andrews and co-workers[12] measured the strength of patients, with hemiplegia of a vascular origin, using the Medical Research Council scale. This scale is as follows: 1 – complete paralysis; 2 – flicker of movement; 3 – movement with effect of gravity removed; 4 – movement against gravity; 5 – movement against weak resistance; and, 6 – movement against strong resistance.

Instrumented tests of the muscle strength of stroke patients have been performed with strain gauges, hand-grip dynamometers, hand-held dynamometers, and isokinetic dynamometers. Employing a strain gauge, Saltin and Landin measured knee flexion and extension and ankle dorsiflexion and plantar flexion.[13] They found that knee flexion and extension were significantly weaker on the paretic side. They also noted that knee flexion was weaker than normal on the non-paretic side. In a study that will be discussed in greater detail in the next section of this paper, Tang and Rymer, using a strain gauge, investigated the factors underlying hemiplegic elbow flexion weakness.[14]

With a grip strength dynamometer, Trombly and Quintana demonstrated a significant difference between the grip strength of hemiplegic patients and normals.[15] Using another more versatile device, the hand-held dynamometer, several investigators have measured the strength of numerous muscle groups in hemiplegic stroke patients. Most of the subjects in two recent studies of the reliability of hand-held dynamometery were patients who were hemiplegic following CVAs.[16,17] These studies demonstrated both the intrarater and interrater reliability as good to high, thus raising doubts about Bobath's claim that muscle testing in stroke patients is unreliable.[6] Bohannon and Smith have completed two retrospective investigations of upper extremity weakness in hemiplegic patients. In these studies, the strength (measured by hand-held dynamometry) of the plegic side was found to be less than that of the non-plegic side.[18,19] Strength was unrelated to time since onset,[18] but the strength at discharge from rehabilitation was significantly higher than on admission.[19] Although the strength deficits of eight tested upper extremity muscle groups were shown to differ significantly from one another by an analysis of variance, only the deficits of the shoulder internal rotator and abductor muscles were found by post-hoc analyses to be less than those of any other muscle group.[19] The strength of head turning away from the side of the lesion was found to be reduced by Mastaglia and associates, who used a hand-held myometer (dynamometer) to measure the maximum strength of head turning.[20]

Isokinetic dynamometers provide the advantage of being suitable for testing dynamic, as well as static, force production. According to Hamrin and colleagues, the torque measurements obtained with this instrumentation provide a valid estimate of functional capacity after a stroke.[21] Findings from investigations with isokinetic dynamometers are consistent with those of Saltin and Landin with a strain gauge; that is, both have demonstrated that patients with CVAs have weakness, bilaterally, but that they are weaker on the side contralateral to the CVA. This finding has been reported for the knee[21,22] and the ankle[23] muscles. Consequent to their findings at the ankle, Sjöström and colleagues suggested that "careful functional assessment of both legs of the supposedly hemiplegia patient should be carried out."[23(p.58)]

According to some investigations, the dynamic strength deficits of stroke patients are greater at high speeds of movement than at lower speeds. Watkins and co-workers reported this conclusion, as have Hamrin and associates.[21,22] Knutsson and Martensson have reported that some patients even have difficulty reaching the preset speed of the dynamometer as the speed is increased.[24] Although these findings may be important, they should be interpreted in light of the findings of normal persons who also demonstrate decreased torque production with increased speed.[25,26] This recommendation is supported by a yet to be published report (Bohannon, 1986), in which 27 hemiplegic patients were tested. In that study, he found that the absolute torque was lower at high speeds, but that the relative decrease in torque with increased speed did not differ significantly between the plegic and non-plegic side. Because torque at speeds greater than 30°/sec (60, 120, 180°/sec) were significantly correlated with those at 30°/sec, he interpreted the difficulty that the patients had at moving forcefully at higher speeds to be a function of their weakness.

Hemiplegic patients seem to have greater difficulty generating muscle force with the limbs and joints in some positions than they do with them in others. The synergies reported by Twitchell, Brunnstrom and others[23,24] may be related to this difficulty. Tests with isokinetic dynamometers, however, have revealed that positional weakness may not be isolated to the hemiplegic side; rather, such weakness may be simply the manifestation of normal biomechanical principles. Bohannon, for example, reported knee flexion torque to be greater with the hip flexed than with the hip extended on both the plegic and non-plegic sides of stroke patients.[29] He further reported that the ratio of knee flexion torque with the hip flexed and with it extended did not differ significantly between sides. Sjöström and associates demonstrated similar findings in stroke patients at the ankle and concluded that "placement of the legs within patterns believed to facilitate (0° knee position) or inhibit (90° knee position) extensor motoneurons did not give rise to systematic strength variations different from those of control subjects."[23(p.58)]

FACTORS UNDERLYING STRENGTH DEFICITS

A muscle's force production depends on the number of its motor units recruited, the frequency with which its motor units can be recruited,[30,31] the type of motor units within the muscle,[32] and the size of the muscle fibers within the motor unit.[33] Any change in the capacity to recruit motor units or in the type of muscle fibers in the motor unit may, therefore, influence strength. Factors related to strength deficits following CVAs, that will be discussed, are lesion location, motor unit recruitment, muscle changes, and antagonist restraint.

Lesion Location

The importance of primary motor cortex neurons and their projections to muscle force production[34,35] is now common knowledge. Given this importance, it is only logical that a vascular disruption of the motor cortex or of its descending tracts can influence muscle force production. Several recent findings relevant to the relationship between lesion location and motor deficit follow.

Lundgren and associates have reported that damage to the central brain (thalamus, basal ganglia, and internal capsule) results in a greater motor deficit than does neocortical damage.[36] They did not find lesion size to be overly important as a determinant of residual motor function. Discussing lesion location even more specifically were Stolyarova, Kadykov and Vivilov.[37] They reported considerable recovery in patients with lesions of the thalamic tubercle, posterior segment of the posterior limb of the internal capsule, and the cerebral hemispheres. They reported only slight to moderate recovery from lesions of the anterior segment of the posterior limb of the internal capsule and the white matter of the precentral gyrus.

Lesions in areas not considered as primary loci of motor neurons or their projections can also result in weakness. Freund and Hummelsheim reported that patients with lesions confirmed by computerized tomography to lie anterior to the precentral gyrus (in the premotor cortex) had "moderate unilateral weakness of shoulder and hip muscles."[38(p.697)] Stenvers and co-workers demonstrated weakness in the soleus ipsilateral to cerebellar lesions in cats.[39]

Motor Unit Recruitment

Electromyographic (EMG) monitoring of the muscles of hemiplegic patients has clearly indicated an impaired capacity of the patient to activate paretic muscles. Dietz and Berger found that, while patients balanced with each lower extremity on a separate force platform, the joint movements on the spastic side were damped and the muscle activation decreased.[40] The decrease in EMG activity was correlated with the severity of paresis. Trombly and Quintana measured EMG during finger extension and grasp in stroke patients and found the normalized integrated EMG activity to be lower in patients than in normals.[15] Sahrmann and Norton attributed movement difficulties in stroke patients to decreased and prolonged agonist recruitment.[41] Although total EMG activity is decreased in paretic patients, the EMG/unit force is evidently increased.[15,42] A decreased motor unit firing rate might explain this increased ratio.[42,13] If the rate of firing is diminished sufficiently, a failure of twitches to fuse into a strong contraction could result.[43] With the frequency of motor unit firing diminished and all available motor units recruited, the increased sense of effort reported by stroke patients[44,45] could result.[42]

Muscle Changes

Related to decreased motor unit firing may be changes that occur in the muscle when it is no longer maximally activated. Spastic muscles have been observed to contain atrophied "white" Type II fibers and hypertrophied "red" Type I fibers.[46] As fiber size is determined by the extent to which a muscle fiber is used, the relative hypertrophy of Type I fibers, compared to Type II fibers, may be a consequence of a neuronal activation that is inadequate to stimulate the higher threshold[32] Type II fibers.

Another change noted by EMG in the muscles of stroke patients is that of denervation. Though typically thought to be a consequence of lower motor neuron lesions, denervation has been noted on EMG in both the upper and lower paretic limbs of patients following CVAs. Spaans and Wilts found fibrillation potentials and positive sharp waves in the weak limbs of 20 of 21 hemiplegic patients.[47] Benecke and associates recorded activity consistent with denervation in 78 of the 101 stroke patients they tested.[48] The denervation related activity, which first occurs two to three weeks following the cerebrovascular accident, diminishes as spasticity develops and voluntary activation increases.[47,48]

Antagonist Restraint

Antagonist restraint has been emphasized by Bobath and others as a major cause of movement dysfunction.[6,7] They believe that this restraint underlies much of what would be considered weakness by my definition. Evidence supports that, in some cases, antagonist restraint does influence the total force an agonist can bring to bear on the environment, but not to the extent that some have suggested. As Landau has so aptly stated, "It is the negative symptoms that are disabling . . . no patient complains of being disabled by a hyperactive knee jerk." In other words, weakness, rather than spasticity, is the primary problem.[49(p.218)]

Restraint that does exist can arise from three sources: coactivation, spasticity, and passive elastic elements. The potential contribution of these forces are discussed hereafter.

Mizrahi and Angel concluded that, in one hemiplegic patient they studied, rapid forearm extension was prevented by hyperactivity of the stretch reflex of the elbow flexors.[50] They referred to the activity of the elbow flexors during faster movements as a "braking force." Like Mizrahi and Angel, Knutsson and Martensson reported increased antagonist response at high speeds.[24] The latter researchers, however, concluded that the restraint from spasticity (resistance to passive movements) was minimal. They found that antagonist resistance was greater during active movements, suggesting coactivation. McLellan's findings also point to coactivation of the antagonist to an agonist during active movement in stroke patients.[51] He found that anti-spastic medication reduced the response of a muscle to passive, but not active, lengthening. Sahrmann and Norton, though finding prolonged agonist recruitment (which could result in coactivation at the beginning of a reversal of movement), did not find antagonist stretch reflexes to be a problem.[41] "No concurrent excitation of the triceps musculature" during isometric elbow flexion was found by Tang and Rymer.[42(p.693)] Similarly, Bohannon and associates discovered a significant correlation between elbow flexion strength deficits and elbow flexor muscle spasticity, but not between elbow flexion strength and elbow extensor muscle spasticity (unpublished data, 1985). Dietz and Berger explained that, because leg muscle EMG activity was reduced, the abnormally high force in the triceps surae of spastic patients is the result of passive muscle restraint. The author has used a force gauge to demonstrate in his clinic (unpublished data, 1986) that the passive torque of the ankle of the plegic side is significantly greater than that of the non-plegic side. This finding was in the presence of EMG activity that was at or near zero on the plegic side.

RECOVERY OF STRENGTH

Some factors relevant to the recovery of strength have already been discussed. The following are some physical evaluative findings that are of importance to the later strength of stroke patients. Basically, these findings indicate that those who are affected more severely soon after their strokes will be affected more severely later on in the recovery process.

Andrews and associates reported that recovery extends over the first six months, after which time it is modest, particularly in muscle strength.[12] They reported less recovery of strength in those who were severely, rather than moderately, disabled at three months. They found greater improvement in mobility and independency than in strength. Initial and final manual muscle test scores were found to be significantly related by Logigian and co-workers.[53] Bard and Hirshberg made a similar observation. According to these investigators, the motion eventually realized was associated with the motion noted early in the post-stroke period.[10] Bohannon and Smith have shown, using hand-held dynamometers, a potentially similar finding in a rehabilitation setting.[18] They found that upper extremity strength deficits at discharge were significantly correlated with those of admission (r = .73 to .85), but not with time since onset.

RELATIONSHIP OF STRENGTH TO FUNCTION

The relationship between strength and function in stroke patients is not firmly established, although such a relationship appears to exist. Andrews and associates posited a relationship between strength and neurological recovery, but questioned whether information about strength improvements provides much of an indication of total recovery.[12] Logigian and colleagues, however, found that manual muscle test scores were significantly related to the gross Barthel Functional Index.[53] Several investigators have reported a relationship between strength and gait performance. Knutsson and Richards suggested that, for those patients whose gaits were characterized by decreased muscle activation, training to improve strength, bracing and/or walking aids seem to result in maximum improvements in gait performance.[4] Hamrin and colleagues found a highly significant relationship between the isokinetic knee flexion and extension torques and locomotion in hemiplegic stroke patients.[21] In a study investigating the relationship between the static strength of seven paretic lower extremity muscle groups and gait, Bohannon found the strength of four muscle groups to be significantly related to both the speed and cadence of hemiplegic gait;[54] these were the hip extensors (r = .595/.637), knee flexors (r = .466/.533), ankle dorsiflexors (r = .559/.647) and ankle plantar flexors (r = .465/.502).

SUMMARY

Although the measurement of strength in stroke patients is derided by some as unreliable or inappropriate, others successfully have measured strength using ordinal scales or instrumented tests. As a consequence of strength testing, the effects of lesion location and initial strength deficits on later strength deficits and functional outcome are being clarified. Antagonist restraint from several sources may alter the apparent demonstration of strength in stroke patients, but is not the primary cause of weakness. Decreased motor unit recruitment and, in some cases, denervation-type changes in plegic muscles are probably the main factors underlying weakness in stroke patients.

NOTES

1. Gautier JL, Pullicino P: A clinical approach to cerebrovascular disease. Neuroradiology 27:452-459, 1985
2. Mayhew TP, Rothstein JM: Measurement of muscle performance with instruments. In Rothstein, JM (ed): Measurement in Physical Therapy. New York, NY, Churchill Livingstone, 1985, pp 57-94

3. Schmidt RA: Motor Control and Learning. Champaign, IL, Human Kinetics Publishers, 1982, pp 3-4

4. Knutsson E, Richards C: Different types of disturbed motor control in gait of hemiparetic patients. Brain 102:405-430, 1979

5. Daniels L, Worthingham C: Muscle Testing Techniques of Manual Examination. Philadelphia, PA, W B Saunders Co (ed 3) 1972, p 8

6. Bobath B: Adult Hemiplegia: Evaluation and Treatment. London, England, William Heinemann Medical Books Limited (ed 2) 1978, pp 18-20

7. Davies PM: Steps to Follow: A Guide to the Treatment of Adult Hemiplegia. New York, NY, Springer-Verlag, 1985, p 48

8. Chan CWY: Motor and sensory deficits following a stroke: Relevance to a comprehensive evaluation. Physiotherapy Canada 38:29-34, 1986

9. McDowell F, Louis S: Improvement in motor performance in paretic and paralyzed extremities following non-embolic cerebral infarction. Stroke 2:395-399, 1971

10. Bard G, Hirschberg GG: Recovery of voluntary motion in upper extremity following hemiplegia. Arch Phys Med Rehabil 46:567-572, 1965

11. Demeurisse G, Demol O, Rolaye E: Motor evaluation in vascular hemiplegia. Eur Neurol 19:382-389, 1980

12. Andrews K, Brocklehurst JC, Richards B et al: The rate of recovery from stroke and its measurement. Int Rehabil Med 3:155-161, 1981

13. Saltin B, Landen S: Work capacity, muscle strength and SDH activity in both legs of hemiparetic patients and patients with Parkinson's disease. Scand J Clin Lab Invest 35:531-538, 1975

14. Tang A, Rymer WZ: Abnormal force-EMG relations in paretic limbs of hemiparetic human subjects. J Neurol Neurosurg Psychiatry 44:690-698, 1981

15. Trombly CA, Quintana LA: Differences in responses to exercise by post CVA and normal subjects. The Occupational Therapy Journal of Research 5:39-58, 1985

16. Bohannon RW: Test-retest reliability of hand-held dynamometry during a single session of strength assessment. Phys Ther 66:206-209, 1986

17. Bohannon RW, Andrews AW: Interrater reliability of hand-held dynamometry. Phys Ther, to be published.

18. Bohannon RW, Smith MB: Upper extremity strength deficits in hemiplegic stroke patients: relationship between admission and discharge assessment and time since onset. Arch Phys Med Rehabil, to be published.

19. Bohannon RW, Smith MB: Strength deficits in eight upper extremity muscle groups of hemiplegic stroke patients on initial and discharge assessment. Phys Ther, to be published.

20. Mastaglia FL, Knezevic W, Thompson PD: Weakness of head turning in hemiplegia: a quantitative study. J Neurol Neurosurg Psychiatry 49:195-197, 1986

21. Hamrin E, Eklund G, Hillgren A-K et al: Muscle strength and balance in post-stroke patients. Upsala J Med Sci 87:11-26, 1982

22. Watkins MP, Harris BA, Kozlowski BA: Isokinetic testing in patients with hemiparesis. Phys Ther 64:184-189, 1984

23. Sjöström M, Fugl-Meyer AR, Nordin G, Wählby L: Post-stroke hemiplegia crural muscle strength and structure. Scand J Rehabil Med (Suppl 7) 53-61, 1981

24. Knutsson E, Martensson A: Dynamic motor capacity in spastic paresis and its relation to prime mover dysfunction, spastic reflexes and antagonist coactivation. Scand J Rehab Med 12:93-106, 1980

25. Yates JW, Kamon E: A comparison of peak and constant angle torque-velocity curves in fast and slow-twitch populations. Eur J Appl Physiol 51:47-74, 1983

26. Aniansson A, Sperling L, Rundgren A et al: Muscle function in 75-year-old men and women. A longitudinal study. Scand J Rehab Med (Suppl 9) 92-102, 1983

27. Twitchell TE: The restoration of motor function following hemiplegia in man. Brain 74:443-480, 1951

28. Brunnstrom S: Movement Therapy in Hemiplegia. A Neurophysiological Approach. New York, NY, Harper and Row Publishers, 1970, pp 7-33

29. Bohannon RW: Decreased isometric knee flexion torque with hip extension in hemiparetic patients. Phys Ther 66:521-523, 1986

30. Ashworth B, Grimby L, Kugelberg E: Comparison of voluntary and reflex activation of motor units. J Neurol Neurosurg Psychiatry 30:91-98, 1967

31. Kosarov D, Gydikov A: Dependence of the discharge frequency of motor units in different human muscles upon the level of isometric muscle tension. Electromyogr Clin Neurophysiol 16:293-306, 1976

32. Bagust J: Relationships between motor nerve conduction velocities and motor unit contraction characteristics in a slow twitch muscle of the cat. J Physiol 238:269-278, 1974

33. Edstrom L, Ekblom B: Differences in sizes of red and white fibers in vastus lateralis of musculus quadriceps femoris of normal individuals and athletes. Relation to physical performance. Scand J Clin Lab Invest 30:175-181, 1972

34. Evarts EV, Fromm C, Kröller J et al: Motor cortex control of finely graded forces. J Neurophysiol 49:1199-1215, 1983

35. Cheney PD, Fetz EE: Functional classes of primate corticomotoneuronal cells and their relation to active force. J Neurophysiol 44:773-791, 1980

36. Lundgren J, Flodström K, Sjögren K et al: Site of brain lesion and functional capacity in rehabilitated hemiplegics. Scand J Rehabil Med 14:141-143, 1982

37. Stolyarova LG, Kadykov AS, Vavilov SB: Restoration of impaired motor functions in patients with cerebral hemorrhage in relation to site of lesion. Soviet Neurology and Psychiatry 15:35-42, 1982-83

38. Freund HJ, Hummelsheim H: Lesions of premotor cortex in man. Brain 108:697-733, 1985

39. Stenvers JW, Eerbeek O, DeJong JMBV et al: Motor activity and muscle properties in the hemidecerebellate cat. Brain, 106:601-612, 1983

40. Dietz V, Berger W: Interlimb coordination of posture in patients with spastic paresis. Impaired function of spinal reflexes. Brain 107:965-978, 1984

41. Sahrmann SA, Norton BJ: The relationship of voluntary movement to spasticity in the upper motor neuron syndrome. Ann Neurol 2:460-465, 1977

42. Tang A, Rymer WZ: Abnormal force-EMG relations in paretic limbs of hemiparetic human subjects. J Neurol Neurosurg Psychiatry 44:690-698, 1981

43. Rosenfalck A, Andreassen S: Impaired regulation of force and firing pattern of single motor units in patients with spasticity. J Neurol Neurosurg Psychiatry 43:907-916, 1980

44. Brodal A: Self-observations and neuroanatomical considerations after stroke. Brain 96:675-694, 1973

45. Gandevia SC: The perception of motor commands or effort during muscular paralysis. Brain 105:151-159, 1982

46. Edström L: Relation between spasticity and muscle atrophy pattern in upper motor neuronal lesions. Scand J Rehabil Med 5:170-171, 1973

47. Spaans F, Wilts G: Denervation due to lesions of the central nervous system. J Neurol Sciences 57:291-305, 1982

48. Benecke R, Berthold A, Conrad B: Denervation activity in the EMG of patients

with upper motor neuron lesions: Time course, local distribution and pathogenetic aspects. J Neurol 230:143-151, 1983

49. Landau WM: Spasticity: The fable of a neurological demon and the emperor's new therapy. Arch Neurol 31:217-219, 1974

50. Mizrahi EM, Angel RW: Impairment of voluntary movement by spasticity. Ann Neurology 5:594-595, 1979

51. McLellan DL: Co-contraction and stretch reflexes in spasticity during treatment with baclofen. J Neurol Neurosurg Psychiatry 40:30-38, 1977

52. Dietz V, Berger W: Normal and impaired regulation of muscle stiffness in gait: A new hypothesis about muscle hypertonia. Exper Neurol 79:680-687, 1983

53. Logigian MK, Samuels MA, Falconer J et al: Clinical exercise trial for stroke patients. Arch Phys Med Rehabil 64:364-367, 1983

54. Bohannon RW: Relationship between gait velocity and cadence and the strength of seven lower extremity muscle groups of hemiparetic stroke patients. Physiotherapy Canada, in press

Motor Deficits of Stroke: Interrelationships and Assessment

Pamela W. Duncan, MA, PT

SUMMARY. Stroke patients usually present with three primary motor deficits: (1) abnormal tone, (2) paresis, and (3) loss of selective motor control. In this review I pose questions about the interrelationship of these deficits and discuss current literature on their neurophysiological bases. In addition, methods for measuring the deficits are presented and, finally, an evaluation process is outlined which will help us to understand more clearly how the deficits are related to abnormal motor control.

INTRODUCTION

A cerebrovascular accident will interfere with many functions, some more than others, and rarely does the patient with stroke present with a single problem. Therefore, a thorough examination of a stroke patient includes assessment of medical and social history, cognitive, perceptual and emotional features, communication abilities, and sensorimotor functions. The analysis of each problem must not be carried out in isolation, but integrated as part of the whole. For example, paresis is the most common feature of stroke; yet, assessment of the patient's motor ability may be influenced by alterations in perception, sensation, or cognition. With full realization, therefore, that many other problems may influence the motor performance, this article is limited to a discussion of the assessment of the motor deficits of stroke.

Mrs. Duncan is an assistant professor in the graduate program in physical therapy, Duke University, Durham, North Carolina 27710.

57

Stroke patients usually present with three primary motor deficits: (1) abnormal tone, (2) loss of selective motor control, and (3) paresis. How are these specific deficits related or interrelated? Do they share cause-effect relationships or are they independent variables representing different neurophysiological entities? As clinicians, we have assumed certain relationships and our assumptions have dictated how we evaluate and subsequently treat motor control problems following central nervous system damage. Two of our commonly held assumptions are: (1) weakness is secondary to an overactive antagonist, and (2) abnormal tone causes stereotypical synergies of stroke. The purpose of this article is to discuss the neurophysiological bases of the three motor deficits, suggest methods for measurements of these deficits, and finally outline an evaluation process which will help us to understand clearly how the deficits are related to abnormal motor control.

ABNORMAL TONE

Abnormal tone is a common feature of stroke, but it is not easily defined and it is even more difficult to evaluate objectively. Initially, the muscles may be flaccid, with decreased resistance to passive movement. As recovery occurs, usually there is a gradual increase in resistance to passive movement that is velocity-dependent. In addition, when the patient actively moves, resistance may be noted in the antagonist. Clinically, both of these restraints to movement are called spasticity; their neurophysiological bases, however, are different.

Burke suggests that spasticity is a symptom, not a disease.[1] The current theories on the pathophysiology of spasticity include: (a) a hyperactive stretch reflex (highly disputed by Burke),[2] (b) decreased interneuronal inhibition[3] and (c) hyperexcitability of the alpha motor neuron.[4] In an attempt to differentiate the passive from the active components of spasticity, Lance has restricted the definition of spasticity to "a velocity dependent increase in the tonic reflex with exaggerated tendon jerks resulting from hyperexcitability of the stretch reflex as one component of the upper motor neuron syndrome."[5] Investigations into the relationship of active movement to spasticity reveal that the "spasticity" observed in active movement is not the result of a hyperactive stretch reflex of the antagonist, but rather to abnormal regulation of its motor neuron pool.[6] This abnormal regulation causes prolonged recruitment of the motor units and delayed cessation of antagonist contraction at the end of the movement. Disorders of reciprocal inhibition also contribute to increased resistance during active movement.[7] For example, if a patient is unable to reciprocally flex and extend the elbow, this movement dysfunction may not be a result of a hyperactive stretch reflex in the biceps but rather prolonged recruitment of the biceps motorneurons which prevents reversal into extension.

In this paper, I will differentiate between the spasticity we observe in passive movement (increased resistance to passive movement that is velocity-dependent) and the spasticity observed in active movement (prolonged recruitment of motor neurons, or disturbances of reciprocal inhibition).

Objective evaluation of spasticity and quantification of changes in spasticity present a significant challenge to physical therapists in the clinical setting. Among the methods posed for measuring resistance to passive movement is the Ashworth scale[8] (Table 1). This scale provides a subjective indication of spasticity, but it is of questionable objectivity.[9] The pendulum drop test provides an objective measure of passive restraint in certain muscle groups.[10] The Cybex II isokinetic dynamometer, which incorporates an electrogoniometer and recorder, can be used to perform a pendulum drop test for quadriceps tone assessment:[11]

Table 1: Ashworth Scale for Assessment of Abnormal
Muscle Tone

0 = no increase in tone
1 = slight increase in tone giving a "catch" when there was movement in flexion or extension
2 = more increased in the limb, but easily flexed
3 = considerable increase in tone during movement
4 = the limb is rigid in flexion or extension

1. the patient is positioned in a sitting or supine position on the Cybex table, with leg hanging over edge of table,
2. the patient is stabilized to the table with thigh, pelvis, and trunk straps,
3. the dynamometer input shaft is positioned laterally over the knee's axis of rotation and the shin pad of the dynamometer arm is strapped just proximal to the malleoli,
4. the stylus of the position angle channel is adjusted,
5. the speed of the isokinetic dynamometer is adjusted to 300°/sec.,
6. the patient is instructed to relax completely,
7. the leg is then raised by the examiner until the knee is fully extended,
8. paper speed is set at 25mm/sec,
9. the patient is reminded to relax his leg, which is then dropped by the examiner and,
10. steps 6 through 9 are performed 5 more times (3 trials are to ensure the patient is relaxed and the last 2 trials are recorded).

In normal subjects, the recordings obtained in sequential drops are not significantly different.[12] The normal extremity falls through the available range of motion without constraint and usually demonstrates from 5 to 6 oscillations (Figure 1A). Patients with spasticity often fail to reach 90° of flexion on the first oscillation (Figure 1B) and may actually experience a reversal in the direction of movement. In addition, they have fewer oscillations.

The restraint in the antagonist which occurs during active voluntary movements may be assessed clinically by comparing torque produced during voluntary reciprocal movement to torque produced during undirectional movement. For example, a patient whose primary movement problem is prolonged activation of the quadriceps will produce minimal knee flexor torque during reciprocal movement, (extension/flexion) but will be able to produce significantly more knee flexion torque when he flexes his knee only. This problem will become worse as velocity of exercise increases. A second method of analyzing restraint to active movement is to set the Cybex isokinetic speed selector to 300°/sec and request that the patient extend and flex his knee as

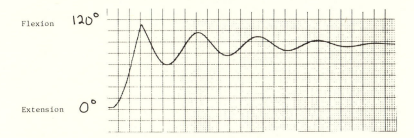

FIGURE 1A. Goniogram of pendulum drop test of uninvolved leg of a 62 year old patient with right hemiplegia. Zero degrees is the initial position of knee extension; the limb freely falls through the available range to approximately 120° of flexion, and the limb then oscillates several times.

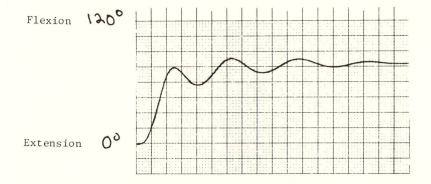

FIGURE 1B. Goniogram of pendulum drop test of involved leg of the same patient as in 1A. The limb does not fall freely and on the initial drop reaches 75° of knee flexion; there are fewer oscillations and less excursion of motion than seen in 1A.

quickly as possible. A patient who has disorders of reciprocal inhibition or prolonged activation of a muscle will not be able to accelerate to 300°/sec and will not be able to flex the knee smoothly without reversing into extension (Figures 2A and 2B).

The goal of clinical assessment is to determine the factors contributing to the "spasticity" syndrome. Resistance to passive movement that is the result of the hyperactive stretch reflex may respond well to drug therapy,[13] physical therapy modalities, slow stretch and/or rotation; but if the problem is abnormal programming of the motor neuron pool for reciprocal movement, the pa-

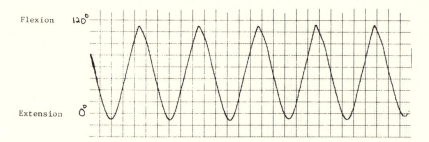

FIGURE 2A. Goniogram of active movement at a velocity setting of 300°/sec on non-involved leg of patient with right hemiplegia. Note that the patient is able to smoothly flex and extend the knee through the available range.

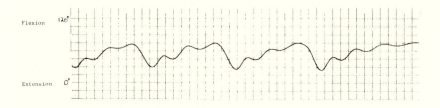

Figure 2B. Active movement at a velocity setting of 300°/sec on involved leg of patient with right hemiplegia. Note that the patient is unable to smoothly flex the knee from an extended position, extends the knee through a limited range of motion, and is unable to achieve the pre-set velocity of 300°/sec.

tient's active movements will not be necessarily improved. Many times, patients with spasticity are treated vigorously to reduce their resistance to passive movement when the latter is not responsible for their active movement deficits. "Under such circumstances, therapy which is effective may not be efficacious."[1]

LOSS OF SELECTIVE MOTOR CONTROL

Many times, the voluntary movement patterns of the stroke patient are limited to the stereotypical flexion and extension synergies described by Twitchell[14] and Brunnstrom[15] (Table 2). These synergies are abnormal in that they are the only degrees of freedom of movement available.[16] Normal movement requires an interweaving of synergies to create an infinite variety of move-

Table 2: Stereotypical Movement Synergies of Stroke as Described by
Brunnstrom

Upper Extremity

Flexor Synergy

Elbow Flexion
Forearm Supination
External Rotation of Shoulder
Abduction of Shoulder
Retraction/Elevation of
   Shoulder Girdle

Extensor Synergy

Elbow Extension
Forearm Pronation
Internal Rotation of Shoulder
Adduction of Shoulder
Protraction of Shoulder Girdle

Lower Extremity

Flexor Synergy

Toe Dorsiflexion
Dorsiflexion and Inversion
   of Ankle
Knee Flexion
Hip Flexion
Hip Abduction & External
   Rotation

Extensor Synergy

Toe Dorsiflexion
Ankle Plantarflexion and
   Inversion
Knee Extension
Hip Extension
Hip Adduction and Internal
   Rotation

ment options. When one or two synergies are the only options for movement, then there is a poverty of movement and a limited repertoire of functional movement patterns.

Spasticity does not cause these stereotypical synergies. The degree of spasticity present and the stereotypical synergies of stroke often wax and wane together. This does not, however, imply a cause-effect relationship. Both spasticity and stereotypical synergies are symptoms of central nervous system damage and they may vary depending on the severity of the brain lesion and the stage of recovery. The loss of selective motor control should be viewed as a disorder of voluntary movement that is due to the malfunction of upper motor neurons centers which participate in the programming and execution of movement, rather than as a result of the spasticity.[17]

The Fugl-Meyer assessment, in which at least 50 different movements are evaluated, is a reliable and valid measure of physical performance following stroke.[18] It objectively measures

degrees of freedom and functional movement patterns independent of any assessment of muscle tone. All movements are
graded on a 3 point ordinal scale (0, unable to perform; 1, perform partially; 2, perform faultlessly). The Fugl-Meyer score has
been shown to correlate well with performance in gait, activities
of daily living, and postural control. The reader is referred to
Fugl-Meyer's original article for specific instructions and guide-
lines for performing this assessment.[18]

PARESIS

Paresis (the inability to produce an appropriate voluntary muscle contraction) is the most salient feature of stroke. Yet, many
clinicians have assumed that paresis is not a primary motor deficit, but rather secondary to an overactive antagonist.[19] The primary motor cortex plays a major role in regulating recruitment
and frequency of motor neuron firing for muscle force production;[20] therefore, paralysis is an expected consequence when the
cortex or the descending motor tracts are disrupted. Several different investigators have demonstrated that, following stroke, the
number of motor units recruited,[21] the type of motor units recruited[22] and the motor unit discharge frequency are altered.[23]
These changes impair force production and increase the effort of
movement. The presence of antagonistic coactivation and of impaired reciprocal inhibition contribute to the paresis but are not
always the primary factor in limiting force production.

The use of manual muscle testing for stroke patients has been
discouraged by many clinicians because of the influence of synergies and spasticity.[15,19] It is true that these factors must be considered; yet, the therapist must be able to assess the patient's
ability to produce force in certain key muscle groups (upper extremity: scapular protractors, shoulder flexors, and abductors,
triceps and biceps, and wrist extensors. Lower extremity: hip
flexors, extensors and abductors, knee extensors and flexors, and
ankle dorsiflexors and plantarflexors). The patient's ability to
produce force repetitively and at different speeds is also a necessary part of the assessment. The ability to produce muscle force
can be evaluated in key muscle groups by using a scoring system
devised by the Medical Research Counsel[24] (Table 3).

Table 3: Medical Research Council
Muscle Grading

0 = no movement or contraction whatsoever.
1 = a palpable contraction, but no movement observed
2 = movement seen at the appropriate joint with
    gravity eliminated
3 = able to move the joint against gravity
4 = able to move the joint against resistance, but
    less than normal side
5 = fully normal power

Isokinetic testing for patients who have recovered the ability to flex and extend the knee against gravity may be used to provide information about the process of force production, power and fatiguability. The following measures can be documented by such testing: (1) peak torque, (2) time to peak torque, (3) limb excursion, (4) velocity-torque relationships, (5) time between reciprocal movement (6), ability to attain and sustain a submaximal torque isometrically, and (7) ability to repeatedly produce torque.[25]

The inability to produce appropriate muscle force is the most disabling motor deficit and should be discretely assessed in stroke patients.

EVALUATION PROCESS

In summary, the motor disorders associated with stroke are extremely complex and are a reflection of the intricacy of normal motor control. Stroke is characterized by a syndrome of motor deficits which may be related but do not necessarily have cause-effect relationships. The most important evaluation that can be performed in a stroke patient is proper clinical evaluation to assess which of the manifestations of the stroke are contributing to the patient's disability. Once these motor deficits have been assessed, their relative contribution to the patient's clinical picture must be evaluated. For example, if the patient has insufficient knee flexion during gait, the therapist first must determine if the patient can generate a muscle force in the knee flexors, then determine if there is active or passive restraint in the quadriceps which would further compromise knee flexion torque, and, finally, must determine if the patient can flex his knee in a variety of functional movement patterns. Through this simple and systematic analysis, the therapist more easily may be able to determine the causes of the movement dysfunction.

NOTES

1. Burke D: Stretch reflex activity in the spastic patient. EEG Suppl 36:172-178, 1982

2. Burke D: Reassessment of the muscle contribution in normal and spastic man. In Feldman RG, Young RR and Koella WP (eds): Spasticity: Disordered Motor Control. Chicago, IL, Year Book Publishers, 1980

3. Delwaide PJ: Human monosynaptic reflexes and presynaptic inhibition: An interpretation of spastic hyperreflective. In Desmedt JE (ed): New Developments in Electromyography and Clinical Neurophysiology. Karger, Basel, Vol 3, pp 508-522, 1973

4. Landau WN: Spasticity: What is it? What is it not? In Feldman RG, Young RR, and Koella WP (eds): Spasticity: Disordered Motor Control. Chicago, IL, Year Book Publishers, 1980

5. Lance JW: Symposium Synopsis. In Feldman RG, Young RR, and Koella WP (eds): Spasticity: Disordered Motor Control. Chicago, IL, Year Book, Medical Publishers, 1980

6. Sahrmann SA, Norton BJ: The relationship of voluntary movement to spasticity in the upper motor neuron syndrome. Annals of Neurology 2:460-465, 1977

7. Miller S, Hammond GR: Neural control of arm movement in patients following stroke. In Van Hof MW, Mohn G (ed): Functional Recovery from Brain Damage. Amsterdam, Elsevier/New Holland, pp 259-274, 1981

8. Ashworth B: Preliminary trial of carisoprodol in multiple sclerosis. Practitioner 192:540-542, 1964

9. Alfieri V: Electrical treatment of spasticity. Scand J Rehabil Med 14:177-182, 1982

10. Vodovnik L, Boyd T: Pendulum testing of spasticity. J Biomed Eng 6:9-16, 1984

11. Bohannon RW, Larkin PW: Cybex II isokinetic dynamometer for the documentation of spasticity. Physical Therapy 65:46-47, 1985

12. King C: Reliability of the pendulum drop test on the Cybex II isokinetic dynamometer. Unpublished Research Project, Graduate Program in Physical Therapy, Duke University, Durham, NC 1986

13. McLellan DL: Co-contraction and stretch reflexes in spasticity during treatment with Baclofen. J Neurol, Neurosurg, Psychiatry 40:30-38, 1977

14. Twitchell TE: The restoration of motor function following hemiplegia in man. Brain 74:443-480, 1951

15. Brunnstrom S: Movement Therapy in Hemiplegia. New York, Harper and Row, 1970

16. Milani Comparetti A: Spasticity vs postural and motor behavior of spastics. Proceedings of the Fourth International Congress of Physical Medicine. New York, Excerpta Medica International Congress Series, No 107, 1964

17. Van Sant A: Designing a definitive clinical study of spasticity. Neurology Report 9:17-19, 1985

18. Fugl-Meyer AR et al: The post-stroke hemiplegic patient: a method for evaluation of physical performance. Scand J Rehabil Med 7:13-31, 1975

19. Bobath B: Adult Hemiplegia: Evaluation and Treatment. London, William Heinemann, 1978

20. Cheney P: Role of cerebral cortex in voluntary movement: A review. Physical Therapy 65:624-635, 1985

21. McComas AJ et al: Functional changes in motoneurons of hemiparetic patients. J Neurol, Neurosurg, and Psychiatry 36:183-193, 1973

22. Mayer RF, Young JL: The effects of hemiplegia with spasticity. In Feldman GR, Young RR and Koella WP (eds): Spasticity: Disordered Motor Control, Chicago, Year Book Medical Publishers, 1980

23. Rosenfalck A, Andreassen S: Impaired regulation of force and firing pattern of single motor units in patients with spasticity. J Neuro, Neurosurg, and Psychiatry 43:907-916, 1980

24. Medical Research Council: Aids to the examination of the peripheral nervous system. Her Majesty's Stationary Office, London 1976

25. Watkins M, Harris BA, Kozlowski BA: Isokinetic testing in patients with hemiparesis: A Pilot Study. Physical Therapy 64:183-189, 1984

Some Aspects of the Causes, Assessment, and Management of the Hemiplegic Shoulder

Sandra C. Brooks, MS, PT

SUMMARY. This paper addresses the causes, evaluation, and treatment of the hemiplegic shoulder, which may be defined as shoulder subluxation, loss of function, and pain, frequently following a cerebrovascular accident. The contribution of the ischemic injury to the brain, prolonged bed rest and immobility, and passive range of motion, traction and compression to the development of this condition is discussed. The importance of an organized approach to assessment and treatment is emphasized.

The "hemiplegic shoulder" connotes subluxation, loss of function, and pain. While 80% of hemiplegic patients experience this problem,[1] its causes are elusive. The neurological damage associated with stroke cannot be solely responsible, as patients with other major neurological insults usually do not encounter this syndrome nor do 20% of hemiplegic patients. The purpose of this paper is to analyze some of the factors leading to the development of the hemiplegic shoulder, to assess such components, and to suggest management strategies to help decrease the negative signs and symptoms.

FACTORS CONTRIBUTING TO THE DEVELOPMENT OF THE HEMIPLEGIC SHOULDER

Since a cerebrovascular accident itself appears not to be the sole etiology of the hemiplegic shoulder, other mechanisms, in-

Ms. Brooks is President of Pediatric Physical Therapy, Inc., 3644 Blaine, St. Louis, MO 63110.

dividually or in concert, also must play a role; a variety of neurological, muscular, and skeletal disorders have been implicated and must be assessed before effective treatment can be initiated.[2,3] For the purposes of discussion, factors influencing the development of shoulder subluxation, pain, and loss of function will be grouped under three categories of events: the ischemic injury to the brain, prolonged bed rest and immobility, and passive range of motion, traction, and compression.

Ischemic Injury to the Brain

The ischemic event, itself, results in muscle weakness, most often a flaccid hemiplegia contralateral to the brain lesion. Because of this weakness and hypotonicity, normal muscular protective responses to stress on the shoulder (e.g., passive range of motion or traction, as in daily care) are lost or ineffective; thus, subluxation may occur because of overstretch of the glenohumeral joint capsule. Additionally, spasticity usually follows the initial flaccid weakness experienced by the patient; spasticity in the scapular adductors and depressors and in the humeral adductors and internal rotators is common and can contribute to soft tissue compression and pain during elevation of the humerus.[4] This is true particularly when attention is not given to proper scapular mobilization and to humeral external rotation. In addition, reports of studies have suggested that, in some stroke patients, shoulder subluxation causes injury to the nerves of the brachial plexus.[3] Such changes may serve as an explanation for prolonged flaccidity and thus affect the prognosis for recovery of function.

Prolonged Bedrest and Immobility

After a cerebrovascular accident, the patient is usually placed on bed rest. This immobility brings changes, particularly in joint and muscle connective tissue, manifested as a decrease or increase in connective tissue flexibility. A decrease in flexibility produces decreased range of motion in the affected joints, particularly the sternoclavicular and acromioclavicular joints. Conversely, an increase in connective tissue flexibility may occur because of overstretching, and this produces excessive range and instability of the glenohumeral joint in particular; for instance, in the supine position gravity may pull the head of the humerus anteriorly and inferiorly. Such overstretching also may occur from kyphotic posture during sitting and weight-bearing; this abnormal alignment and constant stretch may damage the supraspinatus muscle and the shoulder joint capsule, resulting in protective spasm from abnormal compressive forces.

Passive Range of Motion, Traction, and Compression

Direct muscle damage from improper methods of passive range of motion, traction, or compression of the shoulder may result in rotator cuff injuries or tears of the supraspinatus muscle; in such situations, the musculature cannot respond either to support the joint or to contract to actively move the limb. For complete glenohumeral joint abduction to occur without damage to adjacent soft tissue, the scapula must upwardly rotate and the humeral head must depress and externally rotate.

ASSESSMENT AND MANAGEMENT
OF THE HEMIPLEGIC SHOULDER

Methods of assessment of the hemiplegic shoulder range from general observations of the patient's overall posture, and how such posture affects the position of the shoulder, to specific measurements of the shoulder joint complex and the limitation or increase in flexibility of the periarticular structures. The evaluation should be applied methodically, as similar postural and "motor patterns" may have a variety of causes. For example, the classic position of the hemiplegic shoulder may be the result of kyphotic posture, sternoclavicular joint immobility, humeral hyperextension at the glenohumeral joint secondary to an overstretched capsule, spasm or spasticity of the scapular and shoulder musculature, muscle weakness, or combinations of these conditions. A thorough and precise appraisal is mandatory for the establishment of an effective treatment program.

Posture

All related non-shoulder problems, such as kyphotic posture, must be recognized and corrected before the shoulder itself can be assessed and treated. Kyphotic posture may be long standing, as in severe arthritis, secondary to thoracic and lumbar joint flexion from bed rest, or secondary to hip flexion of less than 90 degrees in sitting because of either joint or muscle limitations. The patient may require joint mobilization, stretching, or strengthening of the spine and hip musculature until he can sit and shift his weight forward while keeping the spine extended.

The Shoulder

The degree of mobility of the shoulder girdle joints must be determined before lack of flexibility of the muscles acting on these joints is implicated as a cause of limited joint range of motion. Stretching of muscle tissue, when limited capsular flexibility is the true culprit, may produce abnormal compression of the joint with resulting spasm and pain. Assessment of joint play at the sternoclavicular, acromioclavicular, and glenohumeral joints thus should precede muscle flexibility testing. Frequently, the glenohumeral joint is hypermobile, possibly secondary to hypomobility of the other shoulder girdle joints. If the glenohumeral joint is hypermobile, support to the joint may be needed. A sling may be indicated, but only if it maintains normal joint alignment and if active motion is incorporated into the treatment program.[5]

Assessment of muscle strength should include determination of the amount of joint range against gravity before muscle substitutions are seen, as well as the patient's ability to generate isometric, eccentric, and concentric tension without recruiting activity of synergistic musculature. Strengthening of weakened muscles is critical to overcome effects of disuse and to regain the strength and control of musculature not permanently damaged by the neurological insult.

Malalignment, abnormal joint movement, and pain from damaged structures can all result in muscle spasm. Such spasm, in turn, can cause pain on attempted movement and can limit shoulder mobility. If spasm is contributing to the patient's shoulder problem, deep friction massage or muscle energy techniques, particularly for spasm of the trapezius, serratus anterior, and the rhomboids, may be indicated. In addition, pain may be reduced through the reestablishment of proper shoulder alignment, maintenance of tissue flexibility, and, when possible, the encouragement of active movement.

If active control of shoulder movement does not return after a reasonable time, methods to improve the patient's functional capacity are indicated. The use of adaptive equipment and substitution movements are examples of such an approach.

CONCLUSION

As we have seen, many factors contribute to the development of the "hemiplegic shoulder." Key to the management of patients with this problem is an organized, step-by-step assessment and treatment program, with frequent reassessment of the contribution of each element to the total picture of shoulder subluxation, pain, and loss of function. Such an approach to care allows a variety of treatment options and provides data to document the effectiveness of specific treatment modalities.

REFERENCES

1. Van Ouwenaller C, Laplace PM, Chantraine A: Painful shoulder in hemiplegia. Arch Phys Med Rehabil 67(1): 23-26, 1986

2. Anderson LT: Shoulder pain in hemiplegia. Am J Occup Ther 39 (1): 11-19, 1985

3. Chino N: Electrophysiological investigation of shoulder subluxation in hemiplegics. Scan J Rehab Med 13(1): 17-21, 1981

4. Griffin J, Redden G: Shoulder pain in patients with hemiplegia. A literature review. Phys Ther 61(7): 1041-1045, 1981

5. Smith RO, Okamato GA: Checklist for the prescription of slings for the hemiplegic patient. Am J Occup Ther 35(2): 91-95, 1981